CONTRACEPTION

T0017101

Contraception

The Answers You've Been Looking For

PAULA BRIGGS
Liverpool Women's NHS Foundation Trust

NICOLA KERSEY
Liverpool Community Sexual Health Service

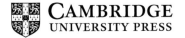

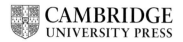

CAMBRIDGE
UNIVERSITY PRESS

Shaftesbury Road, Cambridge CB2 8EA, United Kingdom

One Liberty Plaza, 20th Floor, New York, NY 10006, USA

477 Williamstown Road, Port Melbourne, VIC 3207, Australia

314–321, 3rd Floor, Plot 3, Splendor Forum, Jasola District Centre,
New Delhi – 110025, India

103 Penang Road, #05–06/07, Visioncrest Commercial, Singapore 238467

Cambridge University Press is part of Cambridge University Press & Assessment,
a department of the University of Cambridge.

We share the University's mission to contribute to society through the pursuit of
education, learning and research at the highest international levels of excellence.

www.cambridge.org
Information on this title: www.cambridge.org/9781009124386

DOI: 10.1017/9781009128278

© Cambridge University Press & Assessment 2023

First published 2023

Printed in the United Kingdom by TJ Books Limited, Padstow Cornwall

A catalogue record for this publication is available from the British Library.

A Cataloging-in-Publication data record for this book is available from the Library of Congress

ISBN 978-1-009-12438-6 Paperback

CONTENTS

PREFACE

Women now have more sexual freedom without the risk of pregnancy than at any time in history, often starting in the teenage years and continuing into older age. This means that women are using contraception for much longer than ever before and are better able to plan if and when to have a family. With so much choice and so many misconceptions about contraception, navigating the best option can be difficult. However, it is really important to take time to make the right choice in relation to contraception. Half of pregnancies in the UK are thought to be unplanned. Many women underestimate both the risk of pregnancy, and the life-changing impact of an unplanned pregnancy, irrespective of the outcome.

We wanted to write this book to help women take control of their contraception. Never has there been such a selection with 14 method choices available. Information can be obtained from various sources, including friends, the internet, social media as well as healthcare professionals. However, in the world of social media, where everyone is entitled to an opinion, and misinformation sits alongside valid information, it is no wonder that information can seem conflicting and confusing. Women may be more likely to listen to a friend or an outspoken celebrity than to consider their personal contraceptive needs based on well-researched information. We often see women who switch frequently between methods or suddenly stop using contraception altogether. We also see women who persevere with a method that may not suit them because they are not aware of the alternative options. Many women don't realise that the right method of contraception can contribute to overall well-being. Sex can be enjoyed without concerns about unplanned pregnancy, transmission of sexually transmitted infections is reduced by barrier contraception and common gynaecological problems such as heavy periods can be improved by the use of hormonal contraception. Most importantly, contraception enables women to plan their family.

In this book, we first go back to basics to remind the reader how and when conception can potentially occur during the menstrual cycle. This helps to understand when the risk of pregnancy is highest and when use of contraception is most needed. The two key take-home messages are that anyone who has ovaries and a uterus and has unprotected sex with someone with a penis and testicles is at risk of pregnancy, and that sperm can survive for several days!

We talk about factors that might influence choice and provide a more detailed chapter on each method of contraception. The aim is to provide a framework as the basis for an informed discussion with a healthcare professional about the most appropriate contraceptive choice at the current time of life.

We also aim to dispel many of the myths surrounding contraception: for example, an intrauterine contraceptive, widely known as the coil, is in fact suitable for women of any age, whether or not they have had a baby; the 'morning-after pill' is only effective before ovulation and is not the reliable method of contraception that many believe it to be; hormone treatments for gender reassignment and hormone-replacement therapy during the perimenopause do not provide contraceptive cover.

In writing this book, we hope to empower people of all ages to consider their individual contraceptive choices more carefully and to enjoy their sexual freedom without the fear of an unplanned pregnancy.

INTRODUCTION

The aim of this book is to help women understand what they want from contraception – this may include control of heavy bleeding, for example, in addition to preventing pregnancy – and which options might meet those needs. The aim is not to be too prescriptive – it is a healthcare professional's role to discuss underlying medical issues that might influence the choice of an individual brand of pill, for example. We want women to understand their choices and to feel empowered to have a meaningful discussion with healthcare professionals.

We start the book with a useful reminder of the menstrual cycle because this is fundamental to understanding when and how conception occurs, and therefore why and when contraception is needed. We urge women to read this first chapter, even though they may feel they know about their cycles.

Chapter 2 talks through factors that might influence the choice of contraception, including how different methods might suit women at different stages of their lives and the importance of user factors, such as remembering to take a pill daily compared with a 'fit and forget' method such as the coil. Chapters 3–8 then describe the different methods in more detail: barrier methods (diaphragm, male and female condoms), combined hormonal contraception (the pill, patch and vaginal ring – an underused method, in our opinion), the progestogen-only pill, long-acting reversible contraception (the implant, injection and coil), the fertility awareness method and emergency contraception. The final chapter describes ways in which hormonal contraception can benefit women with a range of gynaecological conditions, such as heavy or painful periods or polycystic ovary syndrome and during the perimenopause.

Chapters 3–8 each start with a summary of the methods discussed in that chapter – how they work, how well they work (effectiveness) and who they are and are not suitable for, so you can quickly see whether the chapter is relevant. Most methods are in fact suitable for most women until about age 50, but how well they work needs to be balanced against a woman's medical history and whether the method will be used correctly. In each chapter we also address common myths that surround contraception, which we hope will help avoid some unplanned pregnancies!

While we are using the term 'woman' in this book, we want to highlight that not everyone with a male body is a man, and not everyone with a female body is a woman. Information in this book is for all genders and non-binary people. Anyone with ovaries, a vagina and a uterus who has unprotected sex with someone with a penis and testicles is at risk of pregnancy. It is a common misunderstanding that gender affirming hormone therapy provides contraception. They don't, and an unplanned pregnancy could be particularly devastating for a trans or non-binary person. However, the long-acting reversible contraceptive methods provide an ideal option for everyone.

There is a lot of information and misinformation in the public domain. We urge readers to check that information they access has been written by suitably qualified experts, and to avoid being unduly influenced by friends and family or social media. People can be quick to complain or to blame contraception for changes such as weight gain or change in libido (sex drive). Misunderstandings and misinformation can be difficult to correct once established; hence, each chapter debunks common myths surrounding contraception.

Each woman is an individual, and what is right for your friend or sister may not be right for you. We hope women will feel informed and able to make their own decisions about the contraception that best suits their health and lifestyle.

1 CONCEPTION AND THE MENSTRUAL CYCLE

In order to understand how to prevent conception, it is helpful to understand when, where and how it happens. Key to this is an understanding of the reproductive system and what happens during the menstrual cycle. This will support understanding of how contraception works. This chapter is a useful overview of the basics, to help with later chapters.

Reproductive Organs

The ovaries have two key functions: they store eggs (ova) and produce the hormones that control the menstrual cycle, reproduction and sexuality. Girls are born with some two million eggs in their ovaries, but the number gradually declines over time; by puberty, typically 250,000 remain. During each menstrual cycle, an egg (ovum) matures in one of the ovaries and is released into the fallopian tube (ovulation). The egg can only be fertilised by a sperm while it is in the first third of the fallopian tube. If fertilisation happens, a blastocyst is created, which is a growing ball of cells that will develop into a fetus.

The womb (uterus) is where a blastocyst implants and grows during pregnancy. The lining of the womb (the endometrium) thickens during the 14 days up to ovulation, in preparation for implantation. Following ovulation, the hormone progesterone released from the egg shell (corpus luteum) causes the number of glands in the lining of the womb to increase, in order to provide nutrients for the blastocyst. If fertilisation doesn't occur, the lining of the womb is shed – this bleeding is a period (menstruation).

The womb is connected to the vagina via the cervix (the neck of the womb), as shown in Figure 1.

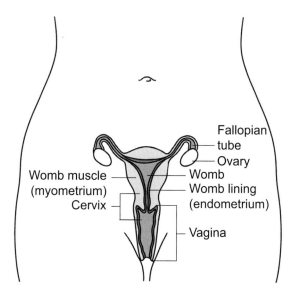

Figure 1 The reproductive organs are contained in the pelvis. The cervix lies between the vagina and the womb. Eggs are stored and develop (mature) in the ovaries and travel along the fallopian tube to the womb.
Artwork © Robin Healy 2022.

The Menstrual Cycle

Day 1 of the menstrual cycle is the first day of bleeding (menstruation – shedding of the lining of the womb). This is also when the next egg starts to develop (mature) in the ovary (so day 1 becomes a more logical designation). Figure 2 shows what happens to the egg and lining of the womb during each cycle.

The Egg

The maturing egg is known as a follicle. It gradually matures during the first 7 days of the cycle. Ovulation occurs around day 13–14 – the egg is released from the follicle into the fallopian tube and

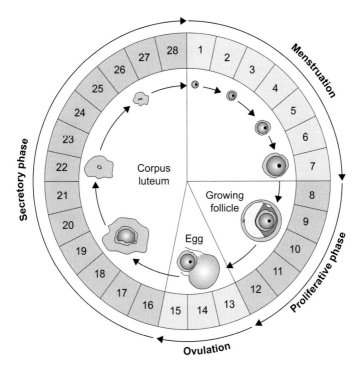

Figure 2 This diagram shows the changes in the womb during the menstrual cycle and the development of the egg. An egg starts to develop (mature) in the ovary while the womb lining is shed during menstruation, and continues through the proliferative stage, which is when the womb lining starts to thicken again. The mature egg is usually released (ovulation around day 13–15). The corpus luteum, which is left behind after ovulation, releases hormones that cause the lining of the womb to thicken and develop glands, in order to support a developing fetus. If the egg is not fertilised, however, the corpus luteum dies and menstruation starts. Drawing adapted, with permission, from artwork by Tetiana Zhabska.

starts to travel towards the womb. The egg leaves a 'shell' in the ovary (the corpus luteum), which releases hormones. In reality, several follicles start to develop, but one generally becomes dominant and capable of releasing a mature egg, with the potential to become a pregnancy if fertilisation occurs.

The Womb

Once menstruation has ended, the lining of the womb starts to thicken again as the follicles develop – this is known as the proliferative phase. Following ovulation, the lining of the womb thickens further and also develops glands that will provide nutrients for a developing blastocyst, if the egg is fertilised. This is known as the secretory phase and predictably lasts 14 days (lifespan of the corpus luteum). If a blastocyst doesn't implant, menstruation starts, marking the start of the next cycle.

Hormonal Control of the Menstrual Cycle

The menstrual cycle is controlled by hormones.

- At the beginning of the cycle, follicle-stimulating hormone (FSH) is released from the pituitary gland in the brain. This triggers growth of the follicles in the ovary, each of which contains an egg (ovum).
- As the follicles develop, they secrete estrogen into the bloodstream. Estrogen causes the lining of the womb to thicken during the first half of the menstrual cycle.
- When the level of estrogen in the bloodstream reaches a critical level, this feeds back to the brain to switch off the release of FSH so that no further eggs mature during that cycle.
- Also, when a critical level of estrogen is reached, another hormone called luteinising hormone is released from the pituitary gland. This triggers the release of the mature egg from the dominant follicle.
- The corpus luteum that remains in the ovary after the egg is released produces both estrogen and progesterone. Progesterone causes the secretory changes in the lining of the womb through its effects on glands, as described above.
- If the blastocyst implants, the corpus luteum continues to produce hormones that support the pregnancy during the first 12 weeks (until the placenta develops and takes over). If implantation does not

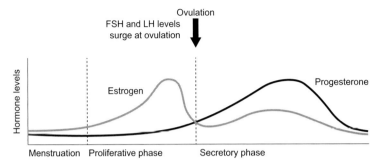

Figure 3 The menstrual cycle is controlled by hormones. Estrogen is released from the developing follicles during the first part of the cycle, so levels rise. Estrogen influences the levels of follicle-stimulating hormone (FSH), which causes the eggs to mature, although, usually, only one is released. Luteinising hormone (LH) triggers release of the egg at ovulation. After ovulation, progesterone is released from the corpus luteum.

occur, the level of progesterone gradually falls and menstruation starts.
- The changes in hormone levels during the menstrual cycle are shown in Figure 3.

Timing of Menstrual Cycles

While the 'average' menstrual cycle lasts 28 days, cycle length varies among women, and also at different times through a woman's reproductive life; cycles of 25–32 days are considered normal. The second (secretory) part of the menstrual cycle predictably lasts about 14 days, whereas the first (follicular) part varies more widely. For example, in a regular 28-day cycle, ovulation occurs at about day 14 and the follicular and secretory stages are each about 14 days. Ovulation occurs earlier in shorter cycles. For example, in a 25-day cycle, menstruation and the follicular stage are likely to last about 11 days while the secretory stage will still be about 14 days, and ovulation is likely to occur at about day 11. This is illustrated in Figure 4.

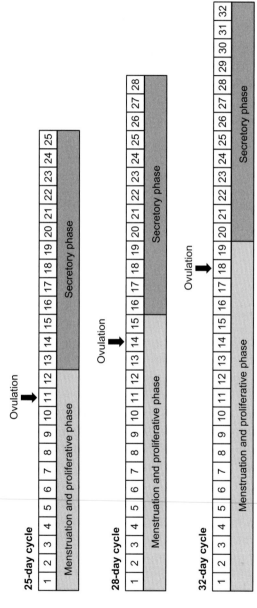

Figure 4 Timing of ovulation in cycles of different length. The secretory phase is predictably 14 days because this is how long the corpus luteum lasts. Women with shorter cycles ovulate earlier than day 14; women with longer cycles ovulate later than day 14. © Helen Barham PhD.

Many women experience irregular cycles, particularly when they first start having periods, and again in later life when they reach the perimenopause, which usually starts from the mid-40s onwards. During these life stages, ovulation does not necessarily occur in every cycle. However, it is important to remember that even when cycles are irregular, ovulation may still occur, so contraception is needed to prevent an unplanned pregnancy. This includes when breastfeeding – many women don't have periods while breastfeeding, but they may still ovulate.

Conception

The term conception refers to implantation, which, in medical terms, is when pregnancy is considered to start. However, some people consider that pregnancy starts at fertilisation – when the sperm and egg combine. The egg survives for no more than 24 hours after ovulation, and the period when fertilisation can occur is just a few hours, when the ovum is in the first third of the fallopian tube (nearest the ovary). However, sperm can survive in the fallopian tubes for several days, so if sperm are already in the fallopian tube at ovulation, fertilisation may occur. This means that the fertile window (i.e., the time when fertilisation is possible) is much longer than the few hours when the egg is viable. If the timing of sexual intercourse, the egg, sperm, fallopian tubes and lining of the womb are all optimal, the chance of achieving a pregnancy in any one cycle is about 25%. Figure 5 shows the most fertile and least fertile parts of the menstrual cycle. While the likelihood of conception varies through the menstrual cycle, contraception should *always* be used to prevent an unplanned pregnancy – for many women there are too many variables to reliably predict a 'safe' time. This is discussed in more detail in Chapter 7.

Contraception – the prevention of conception – can be achieved in three key ways, described in the subsequent chapters:

- by preventing ovulation – this is how the injection, implant and pills work

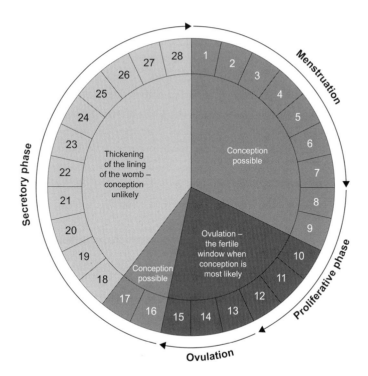

Figure 5 Fertility varies during the menstrual cycle. The most fertile time (which is when conception is most likely) is around ovulation. However, the timing of ovulation is hard to predict, and sperm can live for several days, so there is a risk of conception if a woman has sex without using contraception in the days leading up to ovulation. However, the egg is only viable for 24–48 hours, after which conception is unlikely. © Helen Barham PhD.

- by preventing fertilisation – this is how barrier methods work and methods based on the timing of sexual intercourse
- by preventing implantation – this is how the coil works (in addition, the copper in the copper coil is toxic to sperm, which can prevent fertilisation).

Myth busting: The menstrual cycle and conception

Myth 1: I don't have periods (or my periods are irregular) so I can't get pregnant
> Fact: Even if you aren't having a regular period, you may still be ovulating, for example, when breastfeeding or during the menopause transition – two common misunderstandings.

Myth 2: I am most fertile on day 13/14 of my cycle
> Fact: As shown on Figure 5, you are most fertile *around the time of ovulation*, but this may not necessarily be on day 13/14 – the timing of ovulation can vary. It is also important to remember that sperm can survive for up to 7 days, which extends the fertile window.

Myth 3: You can't get pregnant the first time you have sex
> Fact: You can become pregnant in any menstrual cycle, even if it is the first time you have sex.

Myth 4: You can't get pregnant if you have sex during your period
> Fact: As described above, conception depends on the timing of ovulation and the viability of sperm. Whilst implantation cannot occur while the lining of the womb is being shed during your period, sperm are viable for several days and may therefore survive until you ovulate, particularly if you ovulate early or have a short cycle.

2 MAKING DECISIONS ABOUT CONTRACEPTION

Every sexual encounter (i.e., vaginal penetration with a penis, regardless of whether ejaculation occurs) carries a risk of an unplanned pregnancy unless contraception is used. Women make decisions about contraception throughout their reproductive life, from first sexual activity, through the child-bearing years and then into the perimenopause until the menopause. Some women may quickly find a method that suits them, whereas others will need to try different methods – and may never be truly satisfied. The Contraceptive Counselling (COCO) study of over 1,000 women found that only one-third were very satisfied with their current contraception. One-third were satisfied but wanted to consider a different method, and another third were somewhat satisfied, but felt there might be a more suitable method for them.

It is important that women feel empowered to discuss the full range of contraceptive options with healthcare professionals. This discussion should include the benefits, including non-contraceptive benefits, risks and side effects associated with different methods. It is also important to reconsider contraceptive methods at different stages of life, as needs change and new medical conditions or medication may affect options.

Decisions about the type of contraception to use can be influenced by many factors (Box 1).

This chapter considers issues that may influence decisions about contraception at different stages of life. The later chapters describe the different methods in detail.

The right method of contraception can contribute to overall well-being by:

* supporting an active sex life whilst reducing concerns about unplanned pregnancy

- preventing transmission of sexually transmitted infections (condoms)
- reducing problems associated with periods (e.g., heavy or painful periods)
- being able to plan when to conceive (for personal reasons or because of a pre-existing medical condition)
- planning intervals between pregnancies.

Box 1 Factors that influence decisions about contraception

- Sources of information – from healthcare professionals, leaflets, the internet, social media, word of mouth (e.g., family and friends)
- How well methods work (effectiveness) and how much this depends on the user
- Family planning – is pregnancy planned in the near future?
- Medical history and suitability of different methods
- Implications of pregnancy – how important is it to avoid pregnancy?
- Lifestyle factors
- Sexual activity
- Alcohol or illicit drug taking and how this may affect correct use of certain methods of contraception
- Is it practical to take a tablet daily? Is it easy to remember?
- Menstrual cycle – would there be benefit in regulating or reducing bleeding? (see Chapter 9)
- Additional benefits, such as treating the symptoms of endometriosis or the perimenopause (see Chapter 9)

Accessing Information

Information about contraception can be obtained from many sources: healthcare professionals, patient information leaflets, friends, family, the internet and sex education lessons at school. Use of contraception may be influenced by personal factors such as knowledge and understanding about conception and different methods of contraception, attitudes, perceived risk, family structure and relationships, socioeconomic status, peer influences and access to services.

Knowledge of different methods is important, and choices may be influenced by factors such as effectiveness (how well it works) – and how much this depends on the user – possible side effects, ease of use and how 'invasive' a method is thought to be. Some women may be motivated to take the contraceptive pill reliably every day whereas others may prefer a 'fit and forget' method of contraception, such as the progestogen-only implant or the coil.

Unfortunately, not all sources of information are reliable. However, the wrong information, once accepted, can be difficult to redress – this is what we mean by myths. Many of the myths and misunderstandings relating to contraception are addressed in the individual chapters that follow.

A contraceptive consultation offers a range of additional healthcare benefits, such as screening for sexually transmitted infections (including HIV), vaccinations, cervical screening, health promotion (e.g., help with smoking cessation; management of substance misuse) and support with social issues (e.g., intimate partner violence).

Fertility

In the absence of contraception, the risk of pregnancy depends on the fertility of both partners; the length, regularity and variability of the menstrual cycle; and the timing and frequency of sex.

Fertility is affected by many factors including age, medical conditions, medications, lifestyle factors, such as smoking, and weight. Steps can be taken to improve fertility and the chances of conception; however, irrespective of an individual's medical history, contraception is required by any woman of reproductive age who wants to prevent pregnancy.

Men or women may believe that they are 'infertile' or unlikely to conceive, perhaps because of a medical condition, hormone treatment or because they have not successfully conceived. Nevertheless, even if the risk of conception seems minimal, contraception is important if pregnancy is to be prevented.

Family Planning

Contraception enables individuals and couples to plan when to have a family alongside other life goals such as family commitments, travel, education, a career and achieving financial security. Women are increasingly delaying conception until later in life to achieve an education and career goals before having children. Women also have the opportunity to optimise their health before pregnancy, ensuring good blood-sugar control, weight management and smoking cessation, for example.

Contraception also helps women to plan the interval between pregnancies – for personal as well as health reasons. The World Health Organization recommends a 24-month interval between children. A gap of less than 12 months can be associated with an increased risk of complications, such as preterm labour, stillbirth, low-birth-weight babies and neonatal death.

Other than sterilisation, the use of contraception does not generally compromise longer-term fertility. Fertility returns immediately after stopping contraception with most methods, giving women the flexibility to plan a family. The exception is the progestogen-only injection; fertility usually returns within 6 months, but this can take up to 12 months.

Culture and Trends in Contraception

Contraceptive choice is influenced by a multitude of factors, including cultural issues, education, social and economic factors, religion, fashion and trends. Individual beliefs and ideas about different methods play a large part in method choice.

Women have access to a wide breadth of information and opinions via the internet and social media and increasingly discuss matters with friends and family or via online forums. However, there is a lot of misinformation on social media, including individual 'horror stories' and vocal opinions that may sway individuals. It is important to check that information is from a reputable source, such as the National Health Service in the UK, rather than relying on one individual's experience or agenda – people are quick to report bad experiences but are generally less vocal about good experiences.

It is also important to be aware that pharmaceutical products and devices cannot legally be promoted directly to the consumer in the UK, whereas apps, including natural family planning apps, are not regulated in this way.

Religion and Culture

Organised religions include teaching on sexuality and family formation as fundamental human behaviours and may give guidance on the morality and ethics of sex within and outside of marriage, contraception and abortion, all of which may influence an individual's and couples' attitudes, choices and behaviours. Cultural factors may also influence decisions about family size and when it is acceptable or appropriate to conceive.

Trends

The advent of the contraceptive pill in the 1960s provided women with greater control over their reproductive choices, and had a key role in changing sexual attitudes and freedom; however, the popularity of this method appears to have changed over time in favour of other methods of contraception. These include long-acting reversible contraception – the implant, injection and coil. Natural family planning has received a lot of attention, particularly on social media, portrayed as a 'healthy, natural option'; however, the complexity of this method is usually played down, including the commitment required for success (see Chapter 7). Younger women in particular may be more likely to be influenced by promotional information. However, women are at their most fertile during the early years of their reproductive life, and a more reliable contraceptive method is required to prevent pregnancy.

A contraceptive counselling appointment with a specialist in sexual health or general practice can be helpful to understand the range of options available and to support informed decisions.

When Is Contraception Needed?

Anyone with ovaries and a uterus who has sex with someone with testicles and a penis and who does not want to become pregnant requires contraception, throughout reproductive life (from their first sexual encounter to the menopause). This includes trans-men and non-binary people, even if they are taking masculinising hormones. Sexual activity and contraceptive needs will vary throughout life. For example, a sexually active teenager or young adult may want to avoid pregnancy at all costs, whereas a woman in a stable relationship who is considering having children may be less concerned by an unplanned pregnancy. The imperative not to conceive may increase again later in life, particularly during the perimenopause and once a woman considers that her family is complete.

Many women believe that they cannot conceive if they do not have periods or if their periods are irregular; however, this is not true! Women may still ovulate even if they do not have periods – and the fertile window occurs within 6 days of ovulation. Infrequent ovulation is associated with irregular menstrual bleeding, which can make predicting fertility almost impossible, and a random period may be the first warning that ovulation has already occurred. So, if a pregnancy is not desired, use contraception!

Some women may be advised against pregnancy because of a medical condition, and women and men who are taking certain medications that could harm a developing fetus will be advised to choose an effective method of contraception (ideally one that does not rely on the user) to minimise the risk of an unplanned pregnancy. For women with medical disorders and couples where either partner takes medication that could affect a developing baby, pregnancy should be planned in discussion with their doctors.

Effectiveness of Contraception and Dependence on the User

No method of contraception is 100% guaranteed to prevent pregnancy, but most methods are effective more than 99% of the time. This means that pregnancy is, on average, avoided 99 times out of a 100. Another way to describe this is a failure rate of less than 1% (i.e., no more than one pregnancy among 100 women using the particular method of contraception).

In this book we refer to effectiveness rates for each method of contraception:

- 'Correct and consistent use' refers to perfect use of the method, every time. This includes, for example, taking a pill every day, having injections on time, and using condoms correctly.
- The 'typical use' rates take into account human factors, such as remembering to do something, daily, weekly, monthly or every 12–13 weeks.

Effectiveness rates are higher with correct and consistent perfect use than with typical use, as shown in Table 1. The difference is greater for methods that are highly dependent on the user, such as the pill or condom, and lower for 'fit and forget' methods such as the long-acting reversible contraceptive methods.

How Do I Choose a Method?

Several factors are important when deciding which form of contraception is most appropriate at a particular stage of life. The questions in Box 2 can be helpful in discussions with a doctor, nurse or pharmacist. Options for contraception at different stages of life are discussed towards the end of this chapter.

Contraception for Transgender and Non-binary People

Anyone with ovaries and a uterus who has vaginal sex with someone who has a penis and testicles has the potential to conceive and should therefore use contraception to avoid an unplanned pregnancy.

Non-binary and transgender people often face challenges when discussing contraception with healthcare professionals. However, more sexual health services are providing specialist clinics, and healthcare

Table 1 Effectiveness of different methods of contraception

Method	Effectiveness rate	
	Correct and consistent (perfect) use	**Typical use**
Barrier methods (condoms, diaphragm)	92–98%	79–88%
Combined hormonal contraception (pill, patch, vaginal ring)	More than 99%	91% in first year
Progestogen-only pill	More than 99%	91%
Long-acting reversible contraception (implant, injection, coil)	More than 99%	Implant and coil: 99% Injection: 97%
Fertility awareness method	95–99%	76%
Lactational amenorrhoea method	98%	
Emergency contraception	Coil: 99% Morning-after pill: much less effective than the coil	

'Correct and consistent use' refers to perfect use of the method, every time. This includes, for example, taking a pill every day, having injections on time, and using condoms correctly.

The 'typical use' rates take into account human factors, such as remembering to do something, daily, weekly, monthly or every 12–13 weeks.

The percentages are the number of times the method is effective, so, for example, on average, 92–98 of 100 women using barrier methods will not get pregnant if used consistently and correctly.

Box 2 Questions regarding the most appropriate form of contraception at particular stages of life

---

- How important is it for you to avoid pregnancy at this stage in your life?
- How soon might you want to become pregnant? (e.g., starting or adding to your family)
- How satisfied are you with your current method (if you are using one)? Do you experience any problems?
- How likely are you to use a contraceptive method as intended? (e.g., how likely are you to take a pill every day?)
- What do you want to happen to your periods?
- Do you have any medical issues to consider?
- Are you taking any other medications?
- Is protection against sexually transmitted infections important?

---

professionals are better trained to help. When discussing contraception, it is particularly important to consider current status in terms of hormone use and planned or completed surgery together with any potential risk of sexually transmitted infections. Transgender and non-binary people assigned female at birth (AFAB) may take testosterone therapy or gonadotrophin-releasing hormone (GnRH) analogues. Whilst these suppress ovarian function, they do not provide reliable contraceptive cover. It is also important to be aware that pregnancy must be avoided during testosterone therapy to reduce harm to a developing female fetus.

For AFAB people:

- Progestogen-only methods are not thought to interfere with hormone treatments and have the additional benefit of reducing or stopping vaginal bleeding (these are described in Chapters 5 and 6).
- Long-acting reversible contraception is a good option; the coil that contains the progestogen levonorgestrel may be preferred over the copper coil because they reduce bleeding (these are described in Chapter 6).
- The combined hormonal contraceptive choices (the pill, patch and vaginal ring) are not recommended because the estrogen component may counteract the masculinising effects of testosterone.

Hormone treatments used by transgender and non-binary people assigned male at birth (AMAB), such as estradiol, GnRH analogues, finasteride and cyproterone acetate, reduce but do not inhibit sperm production so contraception is vital if having penetrative vaginal sex.

Sterilisation of either partner is also an option.

Emergency contraception (both oral methods and the copper coil; see Chapter 8) can also be used safely and is not thought to interfere with hormones used by transgender and non-binary people.

A Lifetime of Contraception: From Teenage Years to the Menopause

In this section we discuss how contraceptive needs and decisions may change through a woman's life. Experience demonstrates that women tend to stay with one method of contraception that works for them, and they may not be aware of the wide range of options available, some of which may be more suitable at different life stages.

For this section we have chosen four groups to illustrate the different life stages when the need for contraception and the attitude to a pregnancy may vary:

- young(er) women who are likely to have a strong desire to avoid pregnancy
- women who are ready to plan a family
- women over 40 who do not want to have children, but have yet to reach the menopause
- perimenopausal women.

To make our descriptions easier, we have made some assumptions about women's sexual activity and desire (or not) for pregnancy; however, each person has individual contraceptive needs. When choosing a method of contraception, it is more important to consider the woman's needs, potential benefits, risks and side effects, as well as their attitude to any risk of pregnancy, rather than focusing on age or stage of life. Attitudes to contraception at each stage of life may change over time.

Figure 6 shows how the use of contraception changes with age, based on a survey undertaken in 2009: oral contraception and external condoms are more widely used by younger women, whereas longer-acting methods are more commonly used by older women. However, as

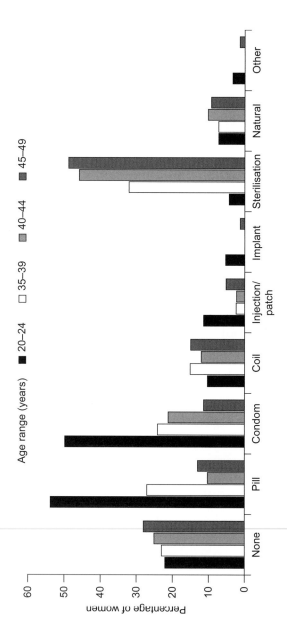

Figure 6 Use of contraceptive methods by women of different age groups. The number of women using long-acting reversible contraception is quite low, despite the benefits. About one-fifth of women of all ages do not use any contraception. Based on data from the Office of National Statistics' 2009 survey on contraception and sexual health.

discussed below, long-acting reversible methods of contraception may be ideal for sexually active younger women, and use of these is increasing. Many young women are not aware that these are potentially good options.

Younger Women

Younger women are more fertile and are at high risk of pregnancy from their first sexual encounter, including before their first period, as ovulation may start before menstruation.

Younger women need support to understand the full range of contraceptive choice, and to feel informed and confident when discussing their contraceptive needs. Sexual health clinicians and most primary care practitioners are comfortable discussing sex, contraception and other personal matters, without being judgemental. Teenagers are likely to be prioritised for appointments in either setting. Confidentiality is ensured (unless sexual abuse, exploitation or terrorism is suspected).

Whilst short-acting contraceptive methods are popular (the pill, the patch or the vaginal ring), their effectiveness depends on the user. The long-acting reversible contraceptive methods may be more suitable for women who want to be sexually active without worrying about an unplanned pregnancy. In order of effectiveness, these are the progestogen-only implant, coil and injection. The long-acting reversible contraceptive methods (the implant, injection, coil) are increasingly being used by this age group; the implant is particularly popular and accepted as the cultural norm.

Women Ready to Start a Family

Women who are ready to start or plan a family have different contraceptive requirements from younger women and they may prefer a method that can be discontinued without medical intervention. However, even with long-acting reversible contraception fertility returns immediately after stopping use (with the exception of the progestogen-only contraceptive injection – it can take 6–12 months for fertility to resume).

Fertility returns 21 days after childbirth, and it is possible for a woman to become pregnant before her first period (ovulation occurs before a period). Women vary in how soon they are ready to have sex after giving birth, but about 50% resume sexual activity within 6 weeks, and many unplanned pregnancies occur during this time. Women are advised to avoid pregnancy for 12–18 months after giving birth, to allow their body to recover and to reduce any risks during the next pregnancy.

It is important to consider postnatal contraception before giving birth and ideally to decide on a method during this time. Waiting until the postnatal check-up at 6–8 weeks is often too late! All the current methods of contraception are suitable following delivery, although the timing differs between methods.

Emergency hormonal contraception (the 'morning-after pill') can be used in the event of unprotected sex from 21 days after childbirth, but the coil can only be fitted after 28 days (see Chapter 6).

Breastfeeding suppresses ovulation and can therefore provide effective contraception (98%) for up to 6 months, as long as the baby is exclusively breastfeeding throughout the day and night and the mother's periods have not started again. This is known as the 'lactational amenorrhoea method' and is described in Chapter 7. The copper in the coil does not affect breastmilk production or quality. Combined hormonal contraception should be avoided in the first 6 weeks following delivery in women who are breastfeeding. Low levels of hormones are excreted in breastmilk and would not harm a baby.

Women over 40

Fertility declines with age, particularly from the mid to late 30s, and pregnancy is rare after 50 years of age. However, the number of women having terminations in their 40s is increasing, possibly because of misunderstanding over pregnancy risk. Contraception is needed until the menopause (see the next subsection) to prevent an unplanned pregnancy.

Decisions by women in this age group may be influenced by similar factors as in younger women, such as motivation to take a pill every day or the desire for a more discrete form of contraception. Long-acting

Table 2 Age-related health conditions that may influence options for
hormonal contraception

Progestogen-only injection	Risks and benefits should be reviewed regularly in women over 40
	A different form of contraception is advised beyond age 50 because of potential effects on bone health
Combined hormonal contraception	Combined pills that contain no more than 30 μg ethinylestradiol are preferred for women over 40 years, because of the potentially lower risk for blood clots, cardiovascular disease and stroke
	Combined pills containing levonorgestrel or norethisterone as the progestogen component are preferred over other formulations because of a potentially lower risk of blood clots
	An estrogen-free method should be used beyond age 50
	The combined pill reduces the risk of ovarian and endometrial cancer; this benefit continues for several decades after discontinuation of the method
	There is a *slight* increase in the risk of breast cancer in women using the combined pill although the absolute rate is very low; there is no significant risk of breast cancer 10 years after stopping treatment
	Women aged 40–50 years can use continuous combined hormonal contraception
	Restarting the combined pill after a break increases the risk of blood clots, so women should not repeatedly interrupt this method of contraception
	Women who smoke should stop combined hormonal contraception at 35 years, when the mortality risk associated with smoking starts to become clinically significant

reversible contraception is popular in this age group, but the specific
contraceptive choice may be influenced by age-related health conditions, such as heart disease, female-specific cancers, bone health and
perimenopausal symptoms (see Table 2).

Barrier methods can be a good option in this age group because declining fertility reduces the risk of pregnancy; however, these methods are user dependent, and effectiveness can be influenced by conditions more common in this age group, such as vaginal prolapse and erectile dysfunction. Natural family planning becomes less reliable as women approach the menopause and, as cycles become less regular, it is increasingly difficult to predict ovulation and the fertile window.

Women may consider sterilisation once their family is complete. However, many methods of contraception are more effective than sterilisation, including the progestogen-only implant and coil, without the risk associated with surgery. Combined hormonal contraception can also potentially help with common gynaecological symptoms such as heavy periods.

Combined hormonal contraception (the pill, patch, vaginal ring) may be appropriate, depending on the individual woman's risk factors, and may help with symptoms of the perimenopause. The vaginal ring may cause an increase in vaginal secretions, which may be a welcome side effect as vaginal dryness can be a problem during the perimenopause! Hormonal contraception that does not contain estrogen does not improve symptoms of the perimenopause such as hot flushes, night sweats and difficulty sleeping.

Some age-related health conditions may influence the choice of hormonal contraception (Table 2). There are no specific health-related concerns with the progestogen-only implant, progestogen-only pill and the coil.

Perimenopause

The perimenopause refers to the years leading up to the menopause, which is defined as 12 months after a woman's last period. During the perimenopause, estrogen levels can fluctuate widely, and menstrual patterns often become erratic. Ovulation no longer happens regularly and bleeding may be unpredictable, heavier and last longer – although in some women periods can stop suddenly.

Hormonal fluctuations experienced at this time can result in a wide range of perimenopausal symptoms. Hot flushes, night sweats, sleep disturbance and mood swings are well-known symptoms, but anxiety, brain fog and joint and muscle aches and pains are less well recognised.

Women aged 50 and older are advised to use contraception for 12 months after their last period (24 months for women under age 50). Women who are using hormonal contraception may not be able to identify when their periods stop and should therefore consider using contraception until 55 years of age. Contraception is no longer needed from age 55 years, as spontaneous conception after this age is exceptionally rare, even in women who still have periods.

Combined hormonal contraception can help to manage perimeno-pausal symptoms, by masking symptoms associated with low and fluc-tuating estrogen levels. However, other health conditions need to be considered when prescribing this type of contraception, particularly in older women. It should be remembered that most hormone-replacement therapy (HRT) does not provide reliable contraception. A 52-mg-progestogen-containing coil can be used for contraception in women of this age group whilst also providing the progestogen com-ponent of HRT (the estrogen component is provided as a pill, patch, gel, spray or implant). If inserted after age 45, the progestogen-containing coil can be left in place until 55 years of age to provide contraception (i.e., for up to 10 years), but it should be changed every 5 years when used as the progestogen component of HRT. The copper coil can remain in place until after the menopause if inserted at age 40 or older.

Summary

Table 3 summarises the recommended contraceptive methods for each life stage, based on our personal clinical experience. Note that most contraceptive methods are suitable for most women.

Table 3 The authors' recommended contraceptive methods at different stages of life

Age group	Recommended methods	
Young women who are likely to have a strong desire to avoid pregnancy	Long-acting reversible contraceptives are the most effective methods Combined hormonal contraception – the pill, patch or vaginal ring	The progestogen-only pill is a good choice for women of any age as long as they are likely to take it correctly
Women who are planning or ready to have a family	Tailored combined hormonal contraception Progestogen-only pill	
Over 40s (i.e., older women who do not want to have children, but have yet to reach the perimenopause)	Contraceptive implant Coil	
Perimenopausal women	Progestogen-containing coil (Mirena®)	

Switching Contraception

Many women find that they need or want to swap to a different form of contraception at different stages in their life – either because their current method is not optimal or because their reasons for using contraception or desire for pregnancy have changed.

It is important to plan the switch to a different type of contraception carefully in order to avoid an unplanned pregnancy. For example, sperm can survive in the fallopian tubes for up to 7 days, so there is a risk of fertilisation if the coil is removed within 7 days of unprotected sex. New methods can take up to seven days to become effective.

Advice from a clinician is recommended when switching between contraceptive methods.

Stopping Contraception

With most methods of contraception, fertility returns immediately when the method is stopped. The exception is the progestogen-only injection (Depot-provera® or Sayana Press®). With both, it can take 6–12 months for fertility to return.

Women may want to stop contraception for various reasons, including times when they are not planning a pregnancy. Some women can be anxious about using hormones for any length of time or think it's a good idea to take a break from hormones, or they may want to see what their natural cycle is like without contraception. However, resuming regular periods does not have any benefit, and the body does not need periods to be healthy. In fact, the absence of periods is beneficial to many women, reducing the risk of anaemia, for example. In addition, periods do not always indicate fertility, and women with irregular or no periods can still ovulate. Women who stop contraception to monitor their periods should be aware of the risk of pregnancy – unplanned pregnancies often occur at these times.

Women who are advised by a specialist to change their contraception should discuss this with the healthcare professional who they consult about contraception in order to avoid an unplanned pregnancy. For example, a surgeon may recommend stopping the pill before undergoing surgery, whereas changing to a non-estrogen method may be appropriate.

Frequent stopping and restarting combined hormonal contraception is not recommended as the risk of blood clots in the legs (deep-vein thrombosis) or lungs (pulmonary embolism) is increased slightly in the first few weeks of use.

Women who want to conceive can stop using contraception at any time and there is no need for periods to be re-established first. A woman may ovulate in her first contraception-free cycle, before her period. Women who need or want to optimise their health, weight or lifestyle before conceiving, or who need to modify medical treatments for established conditions, should continue to use contraception until they are ready to start trying to conceive.

Myth busting: Making decisions about contraception

Myth 1: I'm too old to get pregnant

Fact: It is true that fertility declines with age; however, it is still possible to get pregnant up until the age of 55. Unfortunately, many women believe that, as their periods become less regular, they are no longer fertile. However, they may still ovulate, which means they are at risk of pregnancy. Hormone-replacement therapy does not provide contraception.

Myth 2: The pill is the best contraception for young women

Fact: For young women who have a strong desire not to get pregnant, the patch (changed weekly), vaginal ring (changed every 3 weeks) or long-acting methods (the implant, injection, coil) provide more reliable contraception.

Myth 3: I can just use emergency contraception

Fact: Emergency contraception is not as effective as regular ongoing contraception. In addition, the morning-after pill is only likely to be effective if taken *before ovulation* – for most women this means before day 14 of a 28-day cycle.

Myth 4: I need to stop contraception in plenty of time to allow fertility to return

Fact: Contraception does not affect fertility in the longer term. With the exception of the progestogen-only injection, fertility returns immediately after stopping contraception.

Myth 5: Hormones used by trans and non-binary people prevent conception

Fact: Hormonal medications do not prevent ovulation, so trans and non-binary people who are having this type of treatment are at risk of pregnancy if they have heterosexual sex, even if they are not having periods. In fact, it is important to prevent pregnancy because medications can harm a developing baby.

3 BARRIER METHODS OF CONTRACEPTION

What is it?	Condoms: external (male) and internal (female) Diaphragm: Caya® is the only diaphragm currently in regular use
How is it used?	Barrier methods are put in place before sexual contact, to prevent sperm from coming into contact with a mature egg
How well does it work?	Correct and consistent use: 92–98% Typical use: 79–88%
Who is it suitable for?	Barrier methods are suitable for anyone Condoms are the only method of contraception that protect against sexually transmitted infections All barrier methods are used in conjunction with spermicide
Who is it not suitable for?	People who may forget to use barrier methods, or use them incorrectly Women who need highly effective contraception The diaphragm is not suitable for women with a history of toxic shock syndrome (although this is an exceptionally rare condition) Latex-free (polyurethane) condoms are available

How Do Barrier Methods Work?

These methods prevent fertilisation by creating a physical barrier that prevents sperm from coming into contact with the mature egg (i.e., an ovum capable of being fertilised and developing into a pregnancy).

Additional spermicide is recommended with barrier contraception to increase effectiveness by killing sperm. The individual types of barrier contraception are described in more detail below.

Barrier methods need to be used correctly to be effective, which may be difficult in the heat of the moment! Sperm may be released before ejaculation, so barrier methods should be put in place before any sexual contact. This requires some planning of sex and willingness/awareness to interrupt sex. This may be less likely when couples are under the influence of drugs or alcohol.

Condoms can be used as the sole method of contraception, or at the same time as another method to provide additional protection against pregnancy and sexually acquired infections such as chlamydia and gonorrhoea.

If a barrier method fails for any reason, or there is any doubt about whether it has been used correctly, it might be appropriate to obtain emergency contraception (see Chapter 8).

How Well Do Barrier Methods Work?

As shown in Table 4, barrier methods are 92–98% effective when used consistently and correctly – that is, exactly as intended. However, they

Table 4 Effectiveness of barrier methods of contraception

	Correct and consistent use	Typical use
Male condom	98%	82%
Female condom	95%	79%
Diaphragm + spermicide	92–96%	88%

The values show the number of times out of 100 uses each method would be expected to prevent pregnancy, when used correctly, and with typical use. For example, male condoms, on average, prevent 98 out of 100 pregnancies when used correctly, but only 82 out of 100 pregnancies with typical use.

Correct and consistent use means used exactly as intended; typical use means how the method is used in reality.

are not always used correctly, and they are less effective with typical use – the way they are used in normal life. It is therefore vital to be confident in using barrier methods correctly for *every* sexual encounter, whatever the circumstances.

External (Male) Condoms

How Do They Work?

External condoms are lubricated sheaths that are unrolled onto the erect penis before sex (Figure 7). After ejaculation, semen should remain within the condom, avoiding contact with the woman's genital area. Condoms are available in a range of shapes and sizes (length and width). Latex-free and vegan condoms are also available.

Ensuring Correct Use

The following are key steps to ensure correct use.

- The condom packaging should show safety markings (European conformity (CE) or British Standards Institution (BSI) Kitemark).
- The condom should not be used after the 'use by' date on the packaging.

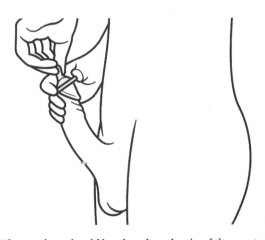

Figure 7 The condom should be placed on the tip of the erect penis, and the teat pinched closed while the condom is rolled down to the base of the penis. The condom should fit tightly, so that it cannot slip or break.
© Dorling Kindersley/Getty Images.

- Care should be taken when opening the packet and removing the condom, to make sure it is not damaged.
- Oil-based lubricants (such as baby oil or petroleum jelly) should not be used, as these can damage condoms made of latex or polyisoprene.
- Lubricant should *not* be used inside the condom, as this may cause slippage.
- The condom should be placed on the tip of the erect penis with the teat facing up and the rim on the outside so that the condom can be rolled down. The teat should be pinched to remove excess air while the rim is rolled down to the base of the penis. If the rim is on the inside, the condom is inside out and should be thrown away and a new one used.
- The condom should fit tightly, so that it cannot slip or break.
- The condom should be applied before the penis comes into contact with a woman's genital region, as sperm can leak from the tip of the penis before ejaculation.
- After ejaculating, the man should withdraw his penis before it goes soft, and remove the condom, keeping it away from the woman's genital area.
- A new condom should be used for each episode of sex.

Internal (Female) Condoms

Internal condoms protect against pregnancy and sexually transmitted infections. They are not widely used but it is good to know they exist!

How Do They Work?

Internal condoms (Figure 8) are lubricated polythene sheaths that are inserted into the vagina before sex. The open end has a larger ring that remains outside the vagina.

Ensuring Correct Use

The following are key steps to improve correct use of internal condoms. It is a good idea to practise inserting the condom, so that is used correctly

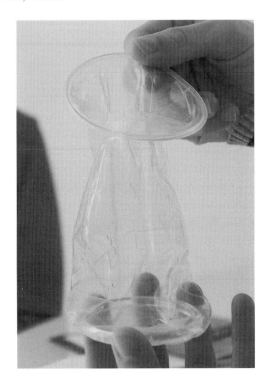

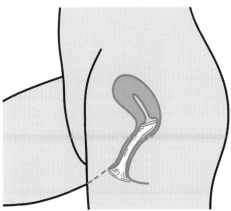

Figure 8 The internal (female condom) is a lubricated polythene sheath that is inserted into the vagina before sex. The open end has a larger ring that remains outside the vagina. Cropped photo © BSIP/ Getty Images. Artwork ©Robin Healy 2022.

during sex. The condom can be put in place up to 8 hours before sex. The following are key steps to ensure correct use.

- The condom packaging should show safety markings (CE or BSI Kitemark).
- The condom should not be used after the 'use by' date on the packaging.
- Care should be taken when opening the packet and removing the condom, to make sure it isn't damaged.
- The ring at the closed (smaller) end of the condom should be squeezed between the thumb and finger and inserted into the vagina, pushing it up as far as it will go. The wider ring must remain on the outside of the vagina (vulva).
- The penis should be guided so that it is inside the condom, not down the side; hold the outer ring in place to ensure that the penis does not go outside the sheath.
- After the penis is removed, twist the outer ring closed and gently pull the condom out and discard.
- Use a new condom for each episode of sex.
- The penis should not come into contact with the woman's genital region without a condom, as sperm may be released before ejaculation.

Diaphragms

Although diaphragms are less commonly used since the advent of other methods of contraception, it is nevertheless useful to be aware of this non-hormonal barrier option. Historically, diaphragms (and caps) had to be fitted by a trained health professional. However, a single-size diaphragm (Caya®; Figure 9) is now available and is suitable for about 80% of women.

It may still be possible to obtain traditional diaphragms in a range of shapes and sizes but these require initial fitting by a trained health professional (although fewer clinicians now have this training).

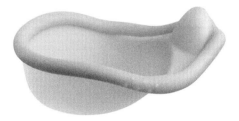

Figure 9 The Caya® single-size diaphragm is contoured and is suitable for about 80% of women. © Medintim.

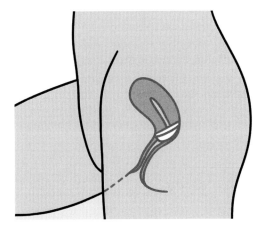

Figure 10 The diaphragm is pushed into the vagina to cover the cervix and area around it, preventing sperm from passing into the womb. It should remain in place for at least 6 hours after sex because sperm can live in the vagina for several hours. Artwork © Robin Healy 2022.

How Do They Work?

The diaphragm is pushed into the vagina with a finger, to cover the cervix and area around it (Figure 10), preventing sperm from passing into the womb. Caya® is provided with a vegan organic spermicide that kills sperm, increasing the effectiveness of the method. If a diaphragm is inserted more than 2 hours before sex, additional spermicide should be applied. The diaphragm should remain in place for at least 6 hours after sex because sperm can live in the vagina for several hours. Latex diaphragms can be left in place for up to 30 hours.

However, additional spermicide must be applied before each episode of sex during this time.

Women with a history of toxic shock syndrome are advised not to use a diaphragm. Diaphragms should not be used while menstruating (i.e., during a period).

Myth busting: Barrier methods of contraception

Myth 1: Condoms are the best and easiest method of contraception

Fact: While condoms can provide effective contraception, they must be used correctly, every time, which can be difficult in the heat of the moment. Other methods that are less dependent on the user may be preferred by women who have a strong desire to avoid pregnancy.

Myth 2: External condoms are unreliable and can break or slip off easily

Fact: External condoms are 98% effective when used correctly and consistently. It is important that condoms are put on correctly every time, and are used all the way through sex (remembering that fluid released from the penis before ejaculation can contain sperm). If a condom is damaged or comes off, emergency contraception is an option. Condoms are the most effective method available to prevent transmission of sexually transmitted infections.

Myth 3: The diaphragm is an old-fashioned contraceptive method

Fact: Whilst diaphragms are used much less nowadays, this can be a useful method of contraception for women who want to avoid hormonal contraception. Caya® is a newer design of diaphragm that fits about 80% of women.

4 COMBINED HORMONAL CONTRACEPTION: THE PILL, PATCH AND VAGINAL RING

What is it?	Hormonal contraception containing estrogen and progestogen
How is it used?	The pill is taken daily for a minimum of 21 days in every 28 Patches are changed once a week for 3 weeks, followed by a patch-free week Vaginal rings are changed every 3 weeks, followed by a ring-free week
How well does it work?	Correct and consistent use: more than 99% effective Typical use: 91% effective in first year
Who are these methods suitable for?	Women who desire flexibility in their contraception The patch and the vaginal ring are ideal for women who prefer not to take a pill daily Women up to age 50 years Women who have painful or heavy periods, or premenstrual disorders
Who are these methods not suitable for?	Women who may not remember to take a pill daily or to change their patch or ring when required Women older than 50 years Women older than 35 years who smoke Women with particular medical conditions, including migraine with aura and a history of blood clots in the leg or the lung Women who are very overweight (body mass index (BMI) 35 kg/m^2 or higher)

Combined hormonal contraceptives contain two hormones, estrogen and a progestogen, which are similar to the body's own hormones. Many people are familiar with the combined oral contraceptive – 'the pill' – but they may not realise that combined hormonal contraception is also available as a patch, changed weekly, and a vaginal ring, which is changed every 3 weeks.

This chapter explains how combined hormonal contraception works and describes the different choices available and the potential health risks for some women. Combined hormonal contraception reduces bleeding and may therefore be a good option for women who have heavy periods (heavy menstrual bleeding) or hormone-related conditions such as polycystic ovarian syndrome and premenstrual disorders. These are described in Chapter 9.

What Is in Combined Hormonal Contraception?

All forms of combined hormonal contraception contain estrogen and a progestogen.

- The estrogen component is usually ethinylestradiol, which mimics naturally occurring estrogen. Modern pills contain 20–35 micrograms of ethinylestradiol, significantly less than the first contraceptive pills introduced more than 50 years ago. The dose of estrogen has been reduced over the decades to limit potential associated health risks. Some newer brands of pill contain 17β-estradiol (which is converted to estradiol – a natural estrogen – in the body) or estradiol instead of ethinylestradiol.
- Progestogens are synthetic hormones that are similar to naturally occurring progesterone. Different progestogens work in slightly different ways and are often described as first-, second-, third- and fourth-generation progestogens (shown in Table 5). The second-generation pills are considered to have the lowest risk of blood clots. Third- and fourth-generation pills were developed to address particular side effects such as acne experienced by some women. A newer pill that contains estradiol and the progestogen nomegestrol acetate (which is similar to natural progesterone) appears to be associated with a similar risk of blood clots as the second-generation pills. It also has fewer side

Table 5 Different generations of progestogens used in combined pills

Generation	Examples	Profile
First	Norethisterone	Some estrogenic effect, which is particularly good for controlling bleeding Not suitable for women who have risk factors for blood clots in the leg/lung (e.g., BMI 30 kg/m^2 or higher)
Second	Levonorgestrel	More potent, so lower doses required
Third	Gestodene, desogestrel, norgestimate (converted to levonorgestrel)	Some estrogen-like effect; increases risk of blood clots in the leg/lung in women with high BMI (30 kg/m^2 or higher)
Fourth	Drospirenone	Prevents fluid retention, which is a side effect of estrogen Blocks the effects of androgens (male hormones that women have at lower levels), which may be helpful for women with facial hair or acne

effects and is thought to be more effective, in preventing pregnancy, particularly in younger women.

How Does Combined Hormonal Contraception Work?

Combined hormonal contraception prevents conception in several ways:

- It prevents ovulation.
- It makes the cervical mucus thicker and more difficult for sperm to penetrate.

- It makes the lining of the womb thinner, so there is less chance that a fertilised egg could implant.

How Well Does Combined Hormonal Contraception Work?

When used correctly and consistently, combined hormonal contraception has a failure rate of less than 1%. However, with typical use, an estimated 9% of women will have an unplanned pregnancy in the first year. Combined hormonal contraception is less effective than long-acting reversible contraception and can fail for various reasons:

- A pill is missed or a new pack is started more than 7 days after the previous pack finished – this is the most common reason for failure.
- The patch or ring is changed later than recommended.
- Absorption of the hormones in the combined pill may be reduced by vomiting and diarrhoea.
- Some medications (including those bought 'over the counter', such as St John's Wort) can cause combined hormonal contraception to be less effective because they increase the rate at which they are broken down (known as liver enzyme-inducing drugs).
- The patch is less effective in women who weigh 90 kg or more.

Fertility returns immediately after stopping combined hormonal contraception. This means that there is an immediate risk of pregnancy unless another contraceptive method is used. Any side effects wear off quickly, as do benefits such as control of bleeding.

Who Can Use Combined Hormonal Contraception?

Combined hormonal contraception can be used until 50 years of age. After this age, the risk factors for cardiovascular disease are considered to outweigh the benefits (see the section on potential risks in Chapter 4) and other methods of contraception should be used (e.g., progestogen-based methods). This form of contraception may not be suitable for women who have particular risk factors or medical conditions (see the section on potential risks below).

How Is Combined Hormonal Contraception Used?

The Combined Pill

The pill is usually used in 28-day cycles: a pill is taken each day for 21 days, followed by a 7-day break (called the hormone-free interval), which induces a 'withdrawal bleed'. When the pill was first developed, the aim was to mimic a natural cycle, with a monthly bleed following withdrawal from the hormones. However, it has become clear that it is safe to take the pill every day without a break, which reduces the risk of forgetting to start on the correct day after the 7-day break. The pill can be taken in a number of different ways, depending on the individual woman's preference, as shown in Box 3. This list is provided to show the broad range of possibilities for using the pill – the best approach – and brand – should be discussed with a clinician.

Ideally, the pill should be taken at about the same time every day; some women keep the pill pack with their toothbrush or another part of a regular morning or evening routine, as a reminder. Pill reminder apps are freely available or reminders can be set on mobile phones. Contraceptive pills are provided in calendar packs so that it is clear which have been taken. The pills should always be taken in the right order.

Box 3 The combined pill can be taken in different ways

- Most brands are taken for 21 days, followed by a 7-day break (the hormone-free interval), resulting in a withdrawal bleed
- Some brands are provided as 'everyday' pills: one pill is taken every day, but only the first 21–24 pills contain hormones; the last 4–7 pills in the packet are placebo (dummy) pills; by taking a tablet every day, women are less likely to forget to start a new packet on time
- Any combined pill can be taken in a tailored way, reducing the hormone-free interval, or can be taken continuously with no hormone-free interval

Missing one pill, or taking it late, is unlikely to increase the risk of pregnancy. The leaflet provided with the pill explains what to do if a pill is missed, depending on when this occurred in relation to the timing of sexual activity. The rules are different for different brands of pill, so it is important to check the instructions for the specific brand being used. Similarly, if looking online for information, it is important to check that the advice is for the particular brand of pill.

The pill may not work properly during periods of diarrhoea or vomiting, or when taking medications that can increase metabolism. Women using the pill should tell any healthcare professional involved in their care what medication they are using and it is a good idea to check the information leaflet in the pill pack. Medication purchased from pharmacies or supermarkets could potentially reduce the effectiveness of combined hormonal contraception.

If there is any doubt about the reliability of contraception after illness, missing a tablet or when taking other medications, an additional form of contraception should be used.

The Patch

Combined hormonal contraception can be delivered as a patch (Figure 11), which releases hormones through the skin into the circulation. The patches are about 4.5 cm square. They are sticky and waterproof, and should stay in place when bathing, showering or swimming.

A new patch is applied once a week for 3 weeks, followed by a 7-day patch-free period (hormone-free interval), during which a withdrawal bleed usually occurs. Patches can also be used continuously (i.e., a new patch every 7 days, with no hormone-free interval) although this may not be stated on the instructions.

The advantages of patches are that they are easy to use and only need to be replaced once a week, rather than taking a pill every day. Some women find this easier to remember, whereas others find a pill taken daily easier to remember. Patches are visible on the skin, which is a helpful reminder (in contrast to a vaginal ring). Unlike the pill, the patch continues to work during illness (sickness or diarrhoea).

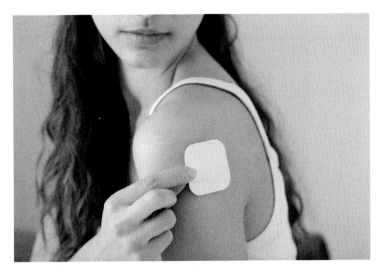

Figure 11 Combined hormonal contraception can be delivered as a patch which releases hormones through the skin into the circulation. The patches are about 4.5 cm square and are waterproof. The patch is worn for 3 weeks, followed by a 1-week gap. Photo © BSIP/ Getty Images.

The patch may continue to provide contraceptive cover if left in place for up to 9 days. The leaflet that comes with the patch explains what to do if the patch has not stuck properly or is starting to come off.

The Vaginal Ring

A soft, plastic ring is inserted to the top of the vagina (Figure 12), in a similar way to a tampon, and slowly releases hormones to provide contraception. It is held in place by the vaginal muscles and is unlikely to come out if it is in the right place, including during sex. The ring does not need to cover the cervix to work (unlike the diaphragm). It is left in place for 21 days, followed by a 7-day ring-free break (hormone-free interval), allowing a withdrawal bleed. However, as with the pill and the patch, the ring can be replaced immediately after 3–4 weeks, without allowing a hormone-free interval.

The advantages of the vaginal ring is that it is easy to use and only needs to be replaced every 3–4 weeks rather than taking

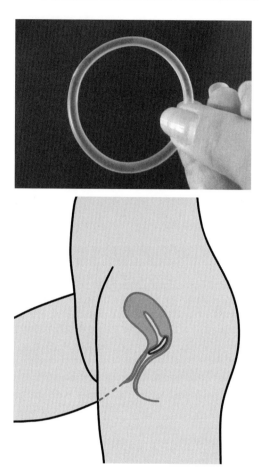

Figure 12 The vaginal ring measures about 5 cm across and is made of flexible plastic. It goes in the same position as the diaphragm (see Figure 10), inserted with a finger, and slowly releases estrogen and a progestogen. It is replaced every 3–4 weeks. Photo © Sandy Huffaker/ Stringer/Getty images. Artwork © Robin Healy 2022.

a pill every day or replacing a patch once a week. Whether this is easier or harder to remember will depend on the user! Unlike the pill, the ring continues to work during illness (sickness or diarrhoea).

The vaginal ring is popular with young people in Europe, but seems to be less popular in the UK. The reason for this is unclear; however, contraceptive methods often go through 'fashions'. The vaginal ring provides good cycle control and works well for women with heavy menstrual bleeding. It is also a good option for women with vaginal dryness (a common perimenopausal symptom), as they increase vaginal secretions. These benefits are explained in more detail in Chapter 9.

Is a Withdrawal Bleed Important?

Withdrawal bleeding during the hormone-free interval is *not* the same as a period. During normal menstrual cycles, the lining of the womb thickens in preparation for a possible pregnancy and is shed if implantation does not happen (i.e., a period). However, when a woman is taking combined hormonal contraception, the lining of the womb does not thicken in the same way, but some blood and mucus is shed during the hormone-free week – withdrawal bleeding.

Withdrawal bleeding is usually lighter and lasts fewer days than a period. However, bleeding can be heavy or painful, and may be associated with headaches and mood changes. Some women find the withdrawal bleed inconvenient. There is also a slight risk that suppression of the ovaries decreases during the hormone-free interval and ovulation may be triggered if pills are missed in the week before or after the scheduled hormone-free interval.

All three types of combined hormonal contraception can be taken continuously for several cycles in order to avoid the hormone-free interval and withdrawal bleeding. Some women worry that they need a monthly withdrawal bleed to be healthy, or that there may be a build-up of menstrual blood if combined hormonal contraception is used without a break. In fact, extended use of this form of contraception keeps the lining of the womb thin. However, continuous use for long periods of time may lead to unpredictable breakthrough bleeding. For this reason, a 4–7-day hormone-free period every 3 months is recommended to help regulate bleeding. Because a shorter hormone-free interval or continuous use of combined hormonal contraception reduces the frequency of withdrawal bleeds and associated symptoms, this approach may help women who have heavy or painful bleeding or problematic symptoms during the hormone-free interval (see Chapter 9).

Side Effects of Combined Hormonal Contraception

All medications have the potential to cause unwanted effects (side effects). Women using combined hormonal contraception have reported headaches, nausea, dizziness and tenderness in the breasts. However, side effects vary between individuals, between products and with the route of administration (the pill, the patch or the vaginal ring). Some side effects occur when starting this form of contraception but improve over 3–4 months. For some women, a shorter hormone-free interval may help reduce side effects. For others, extended or continuous combined hormonal contraception is helpful to reduce symptoms associated with hormone withdrawal, such as headache and mood change.

Overall, it is important not to be swayed by individual reports of side effects, for example on social media, as people can be quick to blame any change in their body (including weight and libido [sex drive]) on medications they are taking, whereas there may be other causes. Based on considerable evidence from clinical trials, combined hormonal contraception does not appear to cause weight gain or loss of libido.

Some women experience irregular bleeding or breakthrough bleeding (i.e., bleeding that is not associated with the withdrawal bleed). It is difficult to predict who might be affected, and changing the brand of pill does not always help. Breakthrough bleeding is thought to decrease over 3–4 months of using combined hormonal contraception. If it continues, an alternative method of contraception may be more appropriate.

While side effects usually get better after 3–4 months, this is not the case for all women. It may be possible to try a different brand of the pill. It is important to discuss changes in contraception with a healthcare professional, to make sure there is not an inadvertent increase in the risk of pregnancy. It is important not to stop and start combined hormonal contraception repeatedly, as this is thought to increase the risk of blood clots (see the next section).

Potential Risks with Combined Hormonal Contraception

While combined hormonal contraception is considered safe for the majority of women, some may have an increased risk of particular health issues such as blood clots. Unfortunately, however, the health risks are often exaggerated or misunderstood by the press and in social media. It is important to understand that the risk of any of these health conditions is very low to start with; a slight increase in risk is still therefore a very low risk. This needs to be balanced against the benefits of combined hormonal contraception and avoiding pregnancy. However, having risk factors does not necessarily mean that this form of contraception should be avoided, but it is important to discuss the advantages and disadvantages with a healthcare professional and to consider alternatives (such as progestrogen-only options; Chapters 5 and 6).

Blood Clots

Venous thromboembolism refers to blood clots that form in the deep veins, most often in the legs (deep vein thrombosis). These clots can travel to the lungs (pulmonary embolism), which can occasionally cause death. The risk of developing a blood clot is increased in women who are overweight (BMI 30 kg/m^2 or higher), who smoke, who are immobile and where there is a family history of clots in close relatives (parents, siblings) below 45 years of age. It is important to recognise that the overall risk of a clot is very low. As shown in Figure 13, it is estimated that 5–10 per 10,000 women of reproductive age will develop a blood clot in any one year. Among those who use combined hormonal contraception, the rate is increased to 7–12 per 10,000 women per year, roughly two additional cases per year. Most women recover from blood clots. Unfortunately, the way that the risk of blood clots has been portrayed in the media in isolation, rather than in a broad context alongside other risks encountered in life, has led to a lot of anxiety. It is important to understand that the risk of clots is significantly higher during pregnancy and after childbirth, and there is a higher risk of death from causes other than blood clots.

The risk of blood clots is greatest during the first few months of using combined hormonal contraception and gradually decreases over a year to

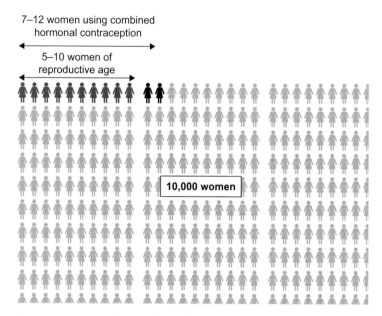

Figure 13 The risk of blood clots when using combined hormonal contraception is very low. Among every 10,000 women of reproductive age, between 5 and 10 are at risk of developing a blood clot. This number increases to 7–12 women using combined hormonal contraception (two additional women in 10,000).

a stable rate. However, the risk is increased again if combined hormonal contraception is restarted after stopping for a month or more, so it is important not to repeatedly stop and restart this form of contraception.

There is some evidence that the risk of blood clots may be slightly higher with the third-generation progestogens compared with the second-generation progestogens (see Table 5). The type and amount of estrogen appears less important, especially with the low doses used in modern combined hormonal contraception.

Cardiovascular Events

The risk of myocardial infarction (heart attack) and stroke is very low in young people but increases with age. The risk in people using combined hormonal contraception is still very low – approximately 3 events per 100,000 individuals in any year.

Many lifestyle and medical factors increase the risk of cardiovascular events (see Box 4), so individuals with any of these conditions may choose a method that does not increase the risk further, usually a method without estrogen. The risks and benefits of combined hormonal contraception should be discussed with a healthcare professional before making a decision – a family history of heart attack/stroke does not mean that a woman cannot use this form of contraception.

Cancer

Use of combined hormonal contraception is associated with a slight increase in the risk of breast cancer and cancer of the cervix. In the case of breast cancer, the risk increases with the duration of use and decreases back to normal over a few years after stopping this form of contraception. Cancer of the cervix is caused by infection with high-risk human papilloma virus infection; the increase in risk seen in women using combined hormonal contraception is likely because they are not using barrier contraception. As with blood clots, it should be remembered that the risk of either type of cancer is very low, and is affected by many factors. On a

---

Box 4 Combined hormonal contraception may not be suitable for all women

Combined hormonal contraception is best avoided by:

- women with high blood pressure (hypertension) that is not controlled with treatment
- smokers over 35 years of age
- women with multiple risk factors for cardiovascular disease, including.
  - smoking
  - high blood pressure
  - high BMI (30 kg/m^2 or higher)
  - abnormal blood lipids
  - diabetes
- women with migraine with aura, or who start getting migraine without aura during combined hormonal contraception use

positive note, women who use combined hormonal contraception have a reduced risk of ovarian cancer and cancer of the womb (uterine cancer).

Myth busting: Combined hormonal contraception

Myth 1: I can't get pregnant if I only miss one pill

Fact: While missing a single pill is unlikely to reduce contraceptive cover, it is wise to take additional contraceptive measures until your next period. Common reasons for failure of the pill include starting a new pack of pills after a break of more than 7 days, and nausea and vomiting, which may reduce its absorption.

Myth 2: My body needs a regular period to be healthy

Fact: Periods do not have any benefit to the body. During normal menstrual cycles, the lining of the womb thickens in preparation for a possible pregnancy and is shed if pregnancy doesn't happen (i.e., a period). Periods return quickly when contraception is stopped.

Myth 3: The pill will make me gain weight

Fact: Based on considerable evidence from clinical trials, the pill does not cause weight gain. People gain weight for many reasons but it is easy to blame the pill!

Myth 4: I'd rather have a copper coil, as hormones are bad for me

Fact: The hormones used in contraception are similar to the body's own hormones, and all current methods use low doses. Use of hormonal contraception can be helpful for common gynaecological problems such as heavy periods (see Chapter 9).

Myth 5: The pill causes blood clots

Fact: The risk of blood clots with the pill has been poorly reported by the media. The risk of blood clots is very low in women in the age range likely to use contraception, and is only slightly increased when taking the pill. Pregnancy and childbirth carry a far higher risk of blood clots.

5 PROGESTOGEN-ONLY PILL

What is it?	A daily pill that contains a progestogen but no estrogen
How is it used?	The POP is taken every day, but to be effective this must be within a 3–24-hour window (depending on the progestogen/brand)
How well does it work?	Correct and consistent use: more than 99% effective at preventing an unplanned pregnancy Typical use: 91% effective at preventing an unplanned pregnancy
Who is it suitable for?	Women up to age 55 years (after which time contraception is not needed) Women who cannot take estrogen
Who is it not suitable for?	Women who may not remember to take a pill within a 3–24-hour window every day (depending on the progestogen)

Chapter 4 talks about combined hormonal contraceptive methods, which contain both estrogen and a progestogen. However, contraception that contains a progestogen alone may be more suitable for women with an increased risk of deep vein thrombosis or cardiovascular disease; this includes women who smoke over the age of 35 and women with a body mass index of 35 kg/m^2 or higher.

This chapter describes the progestogen-only pill (POP). The progestogen-only injection, implant and the coil are described in Chapter 6 on long-acting reversible contraception.

What Does the POP Contain?

The POP contains a progestogen, which is a synthetic version of the hormone progesterone. Newer POPs contain desogestrel or drospirenone whereas older POPs usually contain either norethisterone or levonorgestrel. Desogestrel and drospirenone provide more flexibility in the timing of pill taking (a 12–24-hour window versus 3-hour window – see below).

How Does the POP Work?

The POP prevents conception in several ways.

* It increases the volume and thickness of the cervical mucus, which stops sperm from passing through the cervix into the fallopian tubes. This is the main way in which the older POPs work.
* The POP can prevent ovulation, although this effect differs between the different types of POP: desogestrel and drospirenone stop ovulation most of the time, whereas this is a less reliable effect with the older POPs.
* If ovulation does occur, movement of the egg along the fallopian tubes is slowed.
* The lining of the womb becomes thinner, so that implantation of a fertilised egg is less likely.

How Well Does the POP Work?

The POP is more than 99% effective when used correctly and consistently. However, this requires taking a pill at around the same time every day, which is not easy to do. The POP is 91% effective with typical use.

For older POPs that work mainly by thickening the cervical mucus, this effect is lost if pills are not taken within a 3-hour window. Newer POPs that contain desogestrel or drospirenone need to be taken within a 12–24-hour window to prevent ovulation and therefore tend to be more effective.

Who Can Use the POP?

The POP is suitable for most women and can be taken until age 55 years – when natural fertility is lost. The POP is not thought to increase the risk of heart disease, high blood pressure or breast cancer and it is therefore suitable for women who cannot use combined hormonal contraception because they have risk factors for these conditions.

How Is the POP Taken?

Most POPs are taken continuously every day with no break (i.e., without a pill-free break or hormone-free interval). The drospirenone POP, which is a more recent addition to available choices, is provided in a 24:4 regime, with 24 active pills containing 4 mg drospirenone, followed by four placebo/dummy pills. To be fully effective, these pills should ideally be taken at the same time every day. The POPs available historically were not suitable for women with an unpredictable lifestyle or who are not good at remembering to take pills regularly. This does not apply to pills containing either desogestrel, with a 12-hour window, or drospirenone with a 24-hour window. Use of mobile phone reminders may help, as can taking the pill alongside a regular daily activity such as teeth brushing. The older POPs must be taken within a 3-hour window every day whereas there is a 12–24-hour window for the newer POPs.

Some medications affect the way progestogens are broken down by the body, meaning that POPs may work less well. These drugs are known as liver enzyme-inducing drugs and include some over-the-counter preparations such as St John's Wort. Additional contraception should be used by anyone taking any of these medications for a short period (up to 2 months) and for 4 weeks after stopping the medication. For longer periods it is better to switch to a progestogen-only injection or coil (see Chapter 6). Sickness or diarrhoea may mean that the POP is not absorbed properly, so additional contraception such as condoms is advised during the illness and for 2 days after recovering.

The leaflet provided with the POP explains what to do if a pill is missed, other drugs are being taken and following sickness or diarrhoea. The rules may differ between brands of POP, so it is important to check the leaflet for the specific brand being taken.

The contraceptive effect of POPs is quickly reversible on discontinuation. In addition, POPs are effective within 48 hours of taking the first pill – although the leaflets in the packaging state 7 days before contraceptive cover can be guaranteed.

Side Effects of the POP

Significant changes in bleeding pattern are common with the desogestrel-containing POPs. While the change in bleeding pattern cannot be predicted, bleeding usually reduces gradually, and most women have no bleeding after approximately 12 months of use. A reduction in bleeding is helpful for women who have heavy periods (see Chapter 9). However, if the bleeding experienced during use of a desogestrel POP is troublesome, a healthcare professional should be contacted for help and advice. If no other cause for abnormal bleeding is identified (e.g., infection), a double dose can be tried (under the guidance of a healthcare professional) or initiation of the POP containing drospirenone in a 24:4 regime. The older POPs tend not to cause irregular bleeding as they are less likely to prevent ovulation.

Although some women blame the POP for weight gain, there is no evidence from clinical studies that the POP has this effect.

Myth busting: The progestogen-only pill

Myth 1: It doesn't matter if I miss a pill

   Fact: Because of the way that some POPs prevents pregnancy, it is important that pills are taken at about the same time every day. There is only a 3-hour window with older pills that contain norethisterone or levonorgestrel, whereas there is a little more flexibility with newer POPs that contain desogestrel or drospirenone (12–24 hours).

Myth 2: The POP will make me put on weight

   Fact: Although some women blame the POP for weight gain, there is no evidence from clinical studies that the POP has this effect.

Myth 3: All POPs are the same

   Fact: Different brands of POP are available that contain different types of progestogen.

---

6 LONG-ACTING REVERSIBLE CONTRACEPTION: THE IMPLANT, INJECTION AND COIL

What is it?	The implant and injection slowly release progestogen The coil contains copper or progestogen and is fitted into the womb
How are these methods used?	The implant is inserted under the skin and provides contraception for up to 3 years The injection (sometimes called 'the needle' or 'jag') can be administered by a healthcare professional (Depot-provera®) or self-administered (Sayana Press®); both provide contraception for up to 3 months The coil is fitted inside the womb by a trained healthcare professional and provides contraception for 3–10 years depending on the device
How well do these methods work?	Correct and consistent use: more than 99% Typical use: 99% for the implant and coil; 97% for the contraceptive injection
Who are these methods suitable for?	Women who do not plan to start a family in the immediate future Women who prefer a method that is not user dependent ('fit and forget')
Who are these methods not suitable for?	Injectable contraception may be less suitable for women at risk of osteoporosis

Long-acting reversible contraception has become increasingly popular in place of methods that are dependent on the user, such as oral contraception (both combined and progestogen-only pills). Long-acting methods are highly effective and are suitable for women of any age who do not want to become pregnant in the short term. As well as providing reliable contraception, the hormonal coil can help with common gynaecological symptoms such as heavy menstrual bleeding. This chapter describes the following long-acting methods:

• the implant
• the injection
• the coil.

The Implant

The contraceptive implant is a flexible-synthetic rod about the size of a matchstick (40 mm long; 2 mm wide) that contains the progestogen etonogestrel. It is inserted under the skin (subdermal) in the inner upper arm, usually following administration of a local anaesthetic (Figure 14).

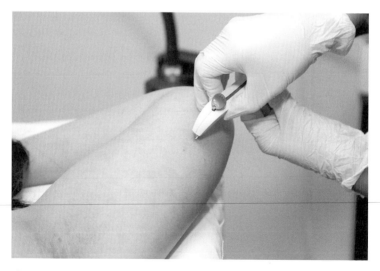

Figure 14 The contraceptive implant is injected under the skin on the inside of the upper arm using a special device, following injection of local anaesthetic to numb the area. Imagedoc/Alamy stock photo.

How Does It Work?

The implant slowly releases etonogestrel into the bloodstream. This hormone is similar to desogestrel in the progestogen-only pill and provides contraception in three ways (in order of importance):

- Ovulation is prevented.
- The lining of the womb becomes thin and inactive, which prevents implantation if fertilisation does occur.
- The cervical mucus becomes thicker, preventing sperm passing beyond the vagina.

This method does not rely on the user and provides contraception for up to 3 years.

How Well Does It Work?

The implant is more than 99% effective and this is the most effective method of contraception available. The contraceptive effect is rapidly reversed after removing the implant, and fertility quickly returns to what is considered normal for the individual.

Some medications (including complementary medications) may affect how well the progestogen works, so, before starting any new medication (including ones bought from a shop or over the counter), it is important to check whether the contraceptive effect of the implant will be affected. This information can be found in the leaflet provided but, if there is any doubt, it is safer to check with a healthcare professional.

Does It Cause Side Effects?

Some women experience prolonged bleeding or spotting when using the implant, whereas other women do not have any bleeding (amenorrhoea). While bleeding is generally reduced, some women find the lack of a predictable pattern difficult to cope with.

Some women experience other side effects such as headache, acne, breast tenderness and mood changes, but these usually settle down after a few months.

The Injection

The contraceptive injection contains medroxyprogesterone acetate, which is injected into a muscle or under the skin every 13 weeks (approximately every 3 months). Injections into the muscle (Depot-provera®) are administered by a healthcare professional whereas injections under the skin (Sayana Press®) can be self-administered after being taught how to do so by a healthcare professional. Both provide contraceptive cover for up to 3 months. Women using the self-injected version can be provided with a year's supply (four uniject devices) reducing the number of visits to sexual health clinics or general practice health centres.

It may take several months (average 6, but up to 12) for ovulation to start again after discontinuing this method of contraception; this should be borne in mind if planning to become pregnant in the near future.

How Does It Work?
The injection works in the same way as the implant:
- Ovulation is prevented.
- The lining of the womb becomes thin and inactive, which prevents implantation if fertilisation does occur.
- The cervical mucus becomes thicker, preventing sperm passing beyond the vagina.

How Well Does It Work?
The injection is more than 99% effective with correct and consistent use (i.e., when the injection is always administered on time). The failure rate is approximately 6% with typical use. This is higher than with other long-acting reversible contraceptives, as the method relies on individuals remembering to have the injection at the correct time.

Does It Cause Side Effects?
All women experience changes in bleeding when using the contraceptive injection and less or no bleeding is likely with longer-term use. Some women – mostly those who are already overweight and younger women – may experience weight gain, which is thought to be because of the effect of the dose of hormone on appetite.

Intrauterine Devices
The coil is a colloquial term referring to an intrauterine device. The coil is a small flexible plastic T-shaped frame (typically about 3 cm wide and

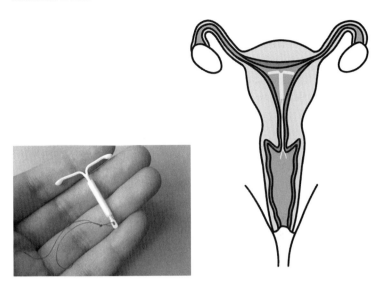

Figure 15 The coil is a small flexible plastic T-shaped frame (typically about 3 cm wide and 3.5 cm long), which contains either copper or a sleeve impregnated with levonorgestrel. The coil is inserted through the cervix into the womb by a trained healthcare professional. The ends of the threads remain on the vaginal side of the cervix, allowing the device to be removed. These threads cannot be felt during sex. Photograph reproduced from Wikicommons under CC SA-BY4.0 licence. Artwork © Robin Healy 2022.

3.5 cm long; Figure 15), which contain either copper or a sleeve impregnated with the progestogen levonorgestrel. The coil is inserted through the cervix into the womb by a trained healthcare professional.

- The coil containing copper can be left in place for up to 10 years (depending on the device).
- The coil containing the progestogen levonorgestrel can be left in place for 3–8 years depending on the type of device and the woman's circumstances.

All currently available devices have threads through the cervix, which the user can usually feel by inserting a finger into the vagina to the cervix. The healthcare professional who fits the device will explain how to check the threads. It is unusual for a woman or for her partner to be aware of the threads during sexual activity.

How Does the Coil Work?

The copper coil releases a very small amount of copper. This prevents pregnancy in several ways:

- Copper is toxic to both the egg and sperm.
- The copper causes an inflammatory reaction in the lining of the womb, which prevents implantation – this is only important if fertilisation occurs.

The progestogen–only coil releases small amounts of the progestogen levonorgestrel into the womb. This provides contraception in two ways:

- The cervical mucus becomes thicker, preventing sperm from passing into the womb.
- The lining of the uterus becomes thinner, which prevents implantation.

Most women continue to ovulate while using this type of coil, but fertilisation and implantation are unlikely.

Several different brands of progestogen-only coils are available in the UK; they provide contraceptive cover for 3–8 years, depending on the brand. Some are also used in hormone-replacement therapy or to manage heavy periods.

How Well Does the Coil Work?

Both types of coil are among the most effective forms of contraception available – they are more than 99% effective. It is important to check regularly that the threads can be felt, to make sure that the device is in the correct place.

Is Insertion and Removal of the Coil Painful?

Insertion of the coil usually takes less than five minutes. It can be uncomfortable, but this does not last long and can be managed with painkillers or, occasionally, local anaesthetic. Some women get cramping (like period pains) afterwards, which can also be managed with painkillers such as paracetamol.

The coil should only be removed by a trained healthcare professional. This procedure is quick and is usually less uncomfortable than insertion.

However, removal can be more uncomfortable if the threads are not visible. Insertion and removal can be performed under general anaesthetic if required.

Does the Coil Cause Side Effects?

Some women have heavier, longer or more painful periods in the first few months after the copper coil is inserted. For most women using the progestogen coil, periods become significantly lighter or stop altogether.

Some women experience pain and irregular bleeding with the coil, and there is a possibility of side effects associated with the hormone levonorgestrel, such as skin and hair changes. Side effects are short-lasting in most women.

What Are the Risks with the Coil?

There is a small risk of infection at fitting, and there is also a small risk (about 1 in 20 cases) that the device may be expelled (usually soon after fitting). The clinician fitting the device will explain the risks and how they are managed. Rarely, in 1–2 per 1,000 women, the device works its way through the wall of the womb into the abdominal cavity. Whilst this is the greatest concern to women, the risk is very low. This is known as perforation. It can be partial or complete and is most likely following pregnancy or in women who are breastfeeding.

Women also worry that the device will 'get lost'. This is unlikely but, occasionally, the threads get drawn up into the cervical canal or the womb. If the threads cannot be felt, ask your doctor to arrange an ultrasound scan to check that the device is in the correct place and is therefore providing reliable contraception. If a device has moved into the abdomen or pelvic cavity, it can be removed with keyhole surgery (laparoscopy).

If a woman has a positive pregnancy test with the coil in place, medical advice should be sought as soon as possible, to rule out ectopic pregnancy (a pregnancy growing outside the uterus, most commonly in the fallopian tube). The overall risk of an ectopic pregnancy is not increased in women with the coil – a common myth.

Myth busting: Long-acting reversible contraception

Myth 1: The implant will be visible

Fact: The implant is placed under the skin on the inner side of the upper arm and is not visible in most women; any scar associated with insertion is tiny.

Myth 2: I can't change my mind once an implant has been inserted

Fact: While the implant is designed to be left in place to provide contraception for up to 3 years, it can be removed at any time. On removal, any side effects experienced wear off quickly. Fertility returns straight away, so it is important to use alternative contraception to avoid an unplanned pregnancy.

Myth 3: I want to start a family soon, so the long-acting contraceptives are not for me

Fact: Fertility returns as soon as contraception is stopped with all the long-acting methods except the contraceptive injection, so they can be used until a woman is ready to start trying to conceive. With the progestogen-only injection, fertility usually returns within 6 months, but can take up to 12 months.

Myth 4: The contraceptive injection reduces fertility

Fact: Fertility takes longer to return to normal after the injection than with other long-acting reversible methods of contraception, but there is no long-term effect.

Myth 5: You can only have the coil if you have had a baby

Fact: Almost any woman can have the coil fitted, regardless of their age or whether or not they have had a baby. Some people believe that it is harder or more painful to fit the coil in younger women, but this is not generally the case.

Myth 6: I didn't get on with the pill, so I can't have the progestogen coil

Fact: The progestogen-only coil releases progestogen directly into the womb. Very little is absorbed into the bloodstream so the risk of side effects is much lower than with the pill.

Myth 7: The coil can go missing

Fact: The coil is inserted through the cervix into the womb, leaving threads that can be felt at the cervix with a finger. Sometimes these threads are hard to find, but it is rare for the coil to be expelled from the womb, and very rare that it works its way through the wall of the womb. In most cases where the threads cannot be felt, they can be seen by a clinician after inserting a speculum. If that is not the case, an ultrasound (or occasionally an X-ray) is used to check the location of the coil.

7 FERTILITY AWARENESS METHOD OF CONTRACEPTION

What is it?	The fertility awareness method (FAM; also described as 'natural family planning') involves the close monitoring of fertility indicators; unprotected sex is avoided during the fertile window or barrier methods of contraception are used The lactational amenorrhoea method (LAM) refers to the contraceptive effect of breastfeeding
How well does it work?	Correct and consistent use of FAM: 95–99% effective Typical use of FAM: 76% effective Correct use of LAM: 98% effective
Who is it suitable for?	FAM is suitable for women who are sufficiently informed to track and record fertility indicators every day and who are prepared to accept a risk of pregnancy
Who is it not suitable for?	Women for whom it is imperative not to become pregnant (e.g., for health reasons and those who are taking a medication that might harm a developing fetus) Women with irregular cycles, including perimenopausal women

The fertility awareness method (FAM) is often called 'natural family planning' and is promoted as 'natural' and may therefore appeal to women who have reservations about using hormonal contraception. FAM is often used by couples planning a pregnancy but it can also be used to avoid pregnancy by using contraception or avoiding sex during the fertile window. However, it is a challenging way to achieve contraception, requiring motivation, commitment and consistency, all of which influence the popularity of this method. FAM is free and success rates are similar to those seen in women using combined hormonal contraception. Women using FAM should be comfortable with a higher risk of pregnancy than with other methods of contraception. FAM is not suitable for women with irregular cycles or those in whom it is imperative not to become pregnant (e.g., for health reasons or because they are taking medication that might harm a developing fetus). It is important to use barrier methods of contraception (usually condoms) if having sex on fertile days (some couples avoid sex on fertile days).

Websites and social media can make FAM sound attractive and easier to use than it really is. It is important to learn the method from someone who has been trained to teach it.

How Does FAM Work?

FAM relies on a careful monitoring of 'fertility indicators' – changes in the body that help identify the fertile window, which is when conception is most likely to occur. These indicators, described in Table 6, include:

- tracking the menstrual cycle to predict the likely timing of ovulation
- measuring body temperature
- checking the texture and consistency of cervical mucus.

For effective contraception, these indicators are best used in combination – this is called the symptothermal method.

Various commercial fertility monitoring devices have been developed; whilst successful in reducing unplanned pregnancy for some women, these probably have the greatest potential in helping women to plan a pregnancy. Some are not intended for use to support contraception and have not been evaluated for this purpose.

Change in Basal Body Temperature

Temperature is measured with a digital thermometer at the same time every morning, before getting out of bed and after resting for at

Table 6 Fertility indicators: a combination of all three provides the best indication of the fertile window and when to avoid sex

Fertility indicator	How is it used?	Fertile window
Change in basal body temperature	Temperature is measured at the same time every morning using a digital thermometer	An increase of at least 0.2 °C indicates that ovulation has occurred The temperature rise must be seen for 3 days in a row, and the temperature should be higher than the previous six days Contraception is not needed from 3 days after the temperature rise until menstruation
Changes in cervical mucus (Billings method)	Cervical mucus is checked every day	The cervical mucus is sticky and appears white at the start of the fertile window The mucus becomes wet, clear and slippery around ovulation After ovulation, the mucus is thick and sticky; once it has been like this for 3 days, the fertile window has ended
Calendar calculations	The menstrual cycle is monitored for at least 12 cycles; the fertile window is calculated using the shortest and longest cycle lengths over the last 12 cycles The Standard Days Method® recommends that sex is avoided on days 8–19 in cycles that are regularly 26–32 days (this method does not work if any cycle is outside this range)	

least 3 hours. Body temperature increases by at least 0.2 °C following ovulation due to the effect of progesterone produced by the corpus luteum and stays elevated until menstruation. This method therefore reflects when ovulation has occurred, rather than when it is likely to occur, and marks the end of the fertile window – contraception is not needed from 3 days after the temperature rise until menstruation.

Other factors can affect body temperature, such as illness and medications, including paracetamol.

It is important to measure body temperature at the same time every day.

Changes in Cervical Mucus

This method (often called the Billings method) involves monitoring changes in the volume and appearance of the cervical mucus during the menstrual cycle.

- For a few days after menstruation, the vagina feels dry and there are no visible secretions.
- As the follicles in the ovaries start to grow, estrogen levels increase and the cervical mucus becomes stickier and is white.
- As estrogen levels continue to rise, close to ovulation, the mucus becomes more slippery, wet, clear and stretchy (a bit like raw egg white). It also becomes alkaline, which makes it easier for sperm to penetrate. This phase is known as the 'peak period' and this mucus is called 'basic fertile mucus'.
- Once the corpus luteum starts to produce progesterone following ovulation, the cervical mucus becomes thicker and stickier again and it is harder for sperm to penetrate.

Mucus can be checked on underwear or toilet tissue or by feeling the genital area, ideally in the afternoon or evening. This must be done every day. The fertile window starts with the first appearance of cervical mucus and continues until 3 days after the peak period. Sex should be avoided on any day when there is mucus during this fertile window, or contraception should be used. Even the tiniest amount of mucus indicates the potential start of the fertile window, so daily monitoring is vital. As a general rule, if *no* mucus is identified on a particular day *and* on the day before (i.e., there is no mucus on two consecutive days), the risk of pregnancy is low.

The cervical mucus should be monitored through several cycles in order to become familiar with the changes.

Calendar Calculations

This method requires menstrual cycles to be monitored for at least 12 cycles to identify the range of cycle length. Ovulation usually occurs between 12 and 16 days *before menstruation*.

*   The first fertile day is taken as 20 days from the end of the shortest cycle.
*   The end of the fertile window is taken as 10 days from the end of the longest cycle.

For example, if the shortest cycle over 12 months is 26 days and the longest cycle is 32 days (which is the case for most women), the fertile window is from day 6 to day 22, so barrier contraception is required during this period or sex should be avoided. Menstrual cycles should always be monitored, in case a longer or shorter cycle occurs, shifting the fertile window.

Another option is the Standard Days Method®, which was developed after studying large numbers of women. This method defines the fertile window as days 8–19 in women who have cycles of 26–32 days (most women). However, this method does not work if *any* cycle is shorter than 26 days or longer than 32 days (as may occur during the perimenopause, for example).

The Symptothermal Method

FAM is more effective when fertility indicators are used in combination. In the symptothermal method, cervical mucus and basal body temperature are monitored and used alongside calendar counting to identify the fertile window, as shown in Figure 16.

Additional Factors

As well as tracking fertility indicators, other factors need to be considered. For example:

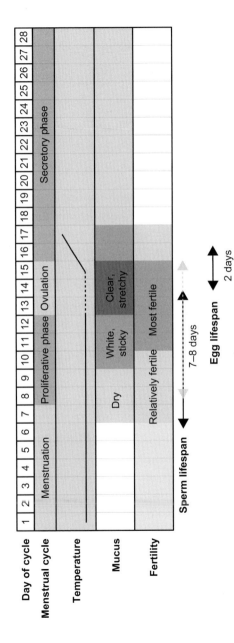

Figure 16 In the fertility awareness method, different methods are combined (calendar calculations, identifying a small increase in temperature, changes in the cervical mucus) to identify the most fertile days of each cycle. Sex is avoided on these days, or barrier contraception used. However, it is important to remember that ovulation is difficult to predict, especially if cycles are irregular. Figure 4 shows the likely timing of ovulation in different length cycles. While the egg is viable for only 12–24 hours, sperm can survive for several days, so it is important that they are not in the fallopian tubes at the likely time of ovulation. © Helen Barham PhD

- body temperature may be affected by infection or illness
- some medications may affect temperature/fertility indicators
- it is easy to become distracted from keeping track of all the necessary elements.

Apps that help women to keep track of their menstrual cycle, temperature and cervical secretions may help improve the effectiveness of FAM for women committed to this method.

How Well Does FAM Work?

The symptothermal method can be as effective as oral contraception when used correctly and consistently: one study reported a pregnancy rate of 0.4% (i.e., 4 in 1,000 women per year) with this method, compared with 0.3% (3 in 1,000) with oral contraception. Another study of 900 women who abstained from sex during the fertile window reported a pregnancy rate of 6 per 1,000 women (0.6%). However, the rate increased to 7.5% when there was sex during the fertile window. The typical pregnancy rate when using only one fertility indicator is about 24%.

The questions posed in Box 5 may help you decide whether FAM is right for you.

Box 5 Is FAM right for me?

- How important is it to avoid pregnancy?
- Do you accept that the risk of pregnancy is relatively high unless the method is followed meticulously?
- Realistically, can you measure body temperature and cervical mucus *every day* and keep track of the changes?
- Do you have regular periods *and* a 12-month record of your menstrual cycles?
- Will you be able to abstain from sex or use a barrier method of contraception on fertile days?

Withdrawal (Coitus Interruptus)

This is *not* considered an effective method of contraception; however, it is included in this book because people need to understand this, especially as it is a popular approach to contraception. This method requires the man to withdraw his penis from the vagina before ejaculating; this means he must be able to recognise when to withdraw, and to commit to doing this, which may prove difficult in the heat of the moment. In addition, the fluid produced before ejaculation may contain viable sperm. Studies suggest failure rates of 4% with correct and consistent use, but 27% with typical use.

Use of the withdrawal method during the fertile window is associated with a high risk of pregnancy and *is not recommended* as a contraceptive method. However, some studies suggest that withdrawal may work when used in combination with FAM.

Lactational Amenorrhoea Method

The lactational amenorrhoea method (LAM) refers to the contraceptive effect of breastfeeding. The ovaries are suppressed by breastfeeding, and women who *fully* breastfeed do not have periods (amenorrhoea) and have reduced fertility for the first 6 months after giving birth. LAM is 98% effective as a method of contraception when *all* the criteria in Box 6 are met.

Box 6 Criteria for LAM to ensure effective contraception – all must be met

- The baby is less than 6 months old
- The mother has not had a period since giving birth
- The baby is exclusively or almost exclusively breastfed
- Intervals between feeds should be no longer than 4 hours during the day or 6 hours at night
- The baby should not be given other liquids/food, other than occasional water

---

It is important to remember that the ovaries are suppressed by breastfeeding, so if the frequency or duration of feeds decrease for any reason, such as illness, the introduction of bottle feeds or the use of dummies/pacifiers, the risk of pregnancy may be increased.

It is not known whether expressing milk (manually or using a breast pump) suppresses ovarian function, so additional contraception will be needed by women who prefer to feed in this way or offer top-up formula feeds.

Myth busting: The fertility awareness method

Myth 1: This an easy method of contraception as I don't have to remember a pill or visit a clinic

Fact: FAM is often promoted as a natural method of contraception (which is true) but, to be effective, this method requires commitment and motivation to measure temperature and cervical mucus *every day* and to keep accurate records of periods for at least 12 months before starting; it is not suitable for women who have irregular periods.

Myth 2: I'm breastfeeding so I can't get pregnant

Fact: Breastfeeding *can* prevent ovulation for the first 6 months after giving birth, but only if the baby is *exclusively* breastfed (no top-up feeds) and the woman does not have any periods. However, lack of periods does not mean that ovulation has not occurred – and ovulation occurs before a period, which may be too late!

Myth 3: The withdrawal method is good enough

Fact: The withdrawal method is not effective, reliable or recommended as a method of contraception because fluid released from the penis before ejaculation may contain sperm.

---

8 EMERGENCY CONTRACEPTION

What is it?	Contraception used soon after unprotected sex to reduce the likelihood of an unplanned pregnancy
	The options are:
	• emergency hormonal contraception (known as the 'morning-after pill', although this term is misleading); there are two types
	• the copper coil
	It is important to contact a healthcare professional as soon as possible to see which method is most suitable
How is it used?	The morning-after pill is taken once, but it is only effective if taken *before ovulation* – this is a common misunderstanding
	The copper coil can be fitted up until implantation of a fertilised egg (up to day 19 in women who have a regular 28-day cycle) – this is why the copper coil is the more effective method of emergency contraception
How well does it work?	The copper coil is more than 99% effective at preventing pregnancy when used correctly for emergency contraception
	The morning-after pill is less effective than the coil – and may not work at all; this is not widely known!

Who is it suitable for?	Women who have had unprotected sex Women whose contraception has failed (e.g., missed pills; split condom)
Who is it not suitable for?	It should only be seen as a 'backup' in case of failure of a contraceptive method rather than as a regular method of contraception The coil may not be suitable for women with pelvic inflammatory disease, allergy to copper or anatomical abnormalities that prevent fitting

This chapter describes the two available approaches to emergency contraception:

- the copper coil
- emergency hormonal contraception (commonly known as the 'morning-after pill') – there are two types.

The aim of emergency contraception is to prevent fertilisation (emergency hormonal contraception) or implantation (copper coil). Emergency hormonal contraception is more widely available and easier to access (for example from pharmacies); however, the copper coil is much more effective at preventing pregnancy after unprotected sex. This is because emergency hormonal contraception is only likely to be effective before ovulation, whereas the coil can be fitted at any time up to 5 days after ovulation, and left in place for ongoing contraception. The copper coil can be obtained through community sexual health services/genitourinary medicine clinics or some general practices.

The Copper Coil

The copper coil prevents conception in two ways:

- copper is toxic to both the egg and sperm so fertilisation is prevented
- it causes inflammation of the lining of the womb, preventing implantation.

The copper coil is over 99% effective at preventing pregnancy when used correctly for emergency contraception. But to be effective, the copper coil must be inserted within 5 days of unprotected sex or up to 5 days after ovulation. However, the exact timing of ovulation can be difficult to predict with certainty. In women who have a regular 28-day cycle, ovulation occurs on day 13/14, so the copper coil can be fitted to provide emergency contraception up to and including day 19. However, in women who have irregular periods or who have recently used hormones (e.g., contraception), the estimation of ovulation is unlikely to be reliable so insertion of the copper coil may not be appropriate.

The copper coil is suitable for most women except those with pelvic inflammatory disease, allergy to copper or anatomical abnormalities that can prevent fitting. It can be fitted in young women and women who have not had a baby. A woman can choose whether to have the coil removed after her next period, or to keep it in place for ongoing contraception (see Chapter 6).

Emergency Hormonal Contraception: The Morning-After Pill

The morning-after pill prevents or delays ovulation. If it is taken before the surge in luteinising hormone that triggers ovulation (see Chapter 1), it can delay ovulation by 5–7 days, after which any sperm in the womb or fallopian tubes should no longer be viable. The morning-after pill should be taken as soon as possible after unprotected sex, to optimise the chance of delaying ovulation. However, irrespective of how quickly it is taken, it is less effective than the copper coil at preventing an unplanned pregnancy.

There are two different emergency hormonal contraceptives:

*   ulipristal acetate (UPA) 30 mg
*   levonorgestrel 1.5 mg.

UPA is slightly more effective than levonorgestrel (i.e., a slightly better chance of protecting against an unplanned pregnancy), but neither option works once ovulation has occurred.

Many women consider emergency hormonal contraception as a useful 'backup'. However, the morning-after pill may not work that well – it is difficult to estimate just how effective it is because it is impossible to be sure of an individual woman's risk of pregnancy in any one cycle and therefore whether or not she would have conceived without the morning-after pill. The morning-after pill is much less effective than most women believe.

Ulipristal Acetate

UPA is taken as a single 30-mg tablet within 5 days of unprotected sex. If ovulation is delayed rather than inhibited, there is still a risk of pregnancy for the rest of that menstrual cycle (i.e., before the next period) so additional contraception should be used. UPA can be taken more than once in a reproductive cycle.

UPA is less effective if taken with other hormones that block its effects, such as other hormonal contraception. This includes hormones taken in the preceding 7 days, and hormones cannot be taken for the next 5 days.

UPA is not suitable for women with severe asthma, liver or kidney disease. It may work less well in overweight women (body mass index (BMI) 30 kg/m^2 or higher) and if women are taking medications that induce liver enzymes (e.g., rifampicin, phenobarbital, carbamazepine, St John's Wort). UPA may not be suitable for women who are breastfeeding.

Levonorgestrel

Levonorgestrel is taken as a single tablet within 72 hours of unprotected sex. There is some evidence that it may be effective for up to 96 hours (although use after 72 hours is unlicensed).

Levonorgestrel is suitable for most women, although a double dose is recommended for women who have a BMI of 26 kg/m^2 or more or weigh more than 70 kg, or who are taking medication that induces liver enzymes. Levonorgestrel may be taken multiple times during the same menstrual cycle but cannot be taken in the same cycle as UPA. However, a better option would be to start regular hormonal contraception or to have the coil fitted.

When Can Emergency Contraception Be Used?

Emergency contraception is only intended to reduce the risk of pregnancy following unprotected sex, for example, when contraception has not been used or the current contraceptive method is thought to have failed. It is not intended as an alternative to effective regular contraception because it is much less effective.

We know from Chapter 1 that the risk of pregnancy is highest around days 7–14 of the menstrual cycle and that most women are less likely to become pregnant at other times of the cycle. However, ovulation can be unpredictable, and sperm can survive in the reproductive tract for up to 7 days, so emergency contraception should always be considered after unprotected sex at any time in the cycle. This reflects the difficulty of predicting ovulation – it is really only possible to confirm that ovulation has occurred if a woman conceives.

Figure 17 shows when the risk of pregnancy is highest and where the different types of emergency contraception work in a woman who has a regular 28-day cycle.

Some women are surprised to learn that the morning-after pill is only effective if taken *before ovulation* – this is because it works by preventing or delaying ovulation. The copper coil prevents fertilisation *and* implantation and is therefore effective for longer.

The morning-after pill does not harm an established pregnancy (i.e., if implantation has occurred) or if used inadvertently by a woman who is already pregnant. The copper coil cannot be fitted more than 5 days after the predicted timing of ovulation as this could disrupt an established pregnancy.

It is important to note that some women do not have regular periods, so it may be difficult to estimate when ovulation is likely, so it may not be possible to fit the copper coil or to be certain that the morning-after pill has been taken before ovulation.

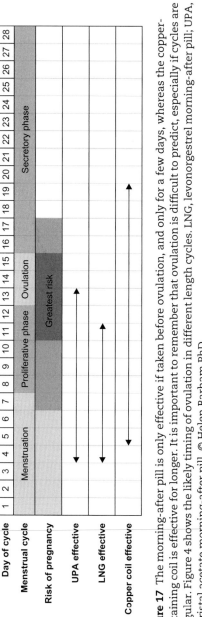

Figure 17 The morning-after pill is only effective if taken before ovulation, and only for a few days, whereas the copper-containing coil is effective for longer. It is important to remember that ovulation is difficult to predict, especially if cycles are irregular. Figure 4 shows the likely timing of ovulation in different length cycles. LNG, levonorgestrel morning-after pill; UPA, ulipristal acetate morning-after pill. © Helen Barham PhD

Myth busting: Emergency contraception

Myth 1: Sperm can be washed out after sex

Fact: Sperm move very fast and can be beyond the cervix within 90 seconds, and only one is required for fertilisation. Washing or douching is therefore unlikely to prevent pregnancy.

Myth 2: The morning-after pill can be taken at any time after sex

Fact: Most people don't realise that the morning-after pill is only effective if taken before ovulation – which may be hard to identify. The coil can be fitted after ovulation to prevent pregnancy.

Myth 3: The coil cannot be fitted in younger women who have not had a baby

Fact: This is a popular myth! The coil can be fitted in women of any age, and regardless of whether or not they have had a baby.

Myth 4: I can just use emergency contraception rather than worrying about other methods

Fact: Emergency contraception is not as effective as many women think. Nor is it as effective as regular contraception – in fact, it is the least effective method of contraception. The morning-after pill must be taken within 3–5 days of unprotected sex (depending on the type) and before ovulation; and the coil can be fitted potentially up to 5 days after the predicted date of ovulation. However, predicting ovulation is difficult. Emergency contraception is not a reliable long-term contraceptive method.

Myth 5: Once I have taken the emergency contraceptive pill, I cannot get pregnant until after my next period

Fact: The emergency contraceptive pill only delays but does not prevent ovulation, and then only if taken at the right time. There is therefore a continued risk of pregnancy with further unprotected sex.

9 USE OF HORMONAL CONTRACEPTION TO TREAT OTHER CONDITIONS

As well as being a valuable form of contraception, hormonal contraception can be used to treat painful periods, heavy periods, premenstrual disorders, acne and polycystic ovary syndrome (PCOS). It can also help to manage symptoms associated with the perimenopause. It is important to consider bleeding patterns and related pain and symptoms when discussing contraceptive choices with healthcare professionals.

Painful Periods

More than half of women experience some pain or cramping during the first one or two days of their period. The pain is caused by chemicals called prostaglandins, which are made in the lining of the womb and make its muscles and blood vessels contract. The level of prostaglandins goes down when bleeding starts, and the pain passes. The pain can usually be managed with painkillers such as ibuprofen and paracetamol. However, about 10% of women experience severe and prolonged cramping pains that can prevent them from doing their normal activities for several days a month. This is known as **primary dysmenorrhoea**. Women may also have other symptoms such as diarrhoea, nausea, vomiting, headache and dizziness.

Girls may experience pain around the time that they start having periods – in fact, this is the most common reason for girls missing school on a regular basis. Periods often become less painful as women get older, and some women notice an improvement following pregnancy.

Women who have fibroids or endometriosis (described below) may also experience painful periods; this is known as **secondary**

dysmenorrhoea, because it is secondary to another condition. The pain usually lasts longer – it may start a few days before a period and continue after it.

Hormonal contraception has been used for many years to treat painful periods when standard painkillers are not enough. Combined hormonal contraception, which contains both estrogen and a progestogen, is most commonly used but progestogen-only methods can also be helpful, such as the progestogen-only pill (POP) containing desogestrel, the progestogen-containing coil, the implant or contraceptive injection – the hormones may prevent ovulation and they thin the lining of the womb.

Combined hormonal contraception works best to reduce painful periods when taken continuously for several months without a hormone-free interval, in order to avoid a withdrawal bleed. Combined hormonal contraceptive choices are described in Chapter 4, the POP in Chapter 5 and long-acting progestogen-only methods in Chapter 6.

Heavy Periods

Some women naturally experience heavy periods, known clinically as heavy menstrual bleeding (HMB). This is often associated with lack of ovulation, as in PCOS, but ovulation can occur spontaneously so contraception is important. As well as being inconvenient, heavy periods may lead to anaemia (low levels of iron in the blood), which can cause tiredness and put health at risk.

Heavy periods may be normal for an individual woman or may have an identifiable cause, such as

- fibroids or polyps
- endometriosis
- hyperplasia (a precursor to endometrial cancer).

These are described in the subsections below.

Fibroids and Polyps

Fibroids (also called uterine leiomyomas) are benign (non-cancerous) growths that develop in and around the womb. They are made up of muscle and fibrous tissue and vary in size – from a pea to a melon. The site rather than the size is more important when considering impact. Fibroids that distort the cavity of the womb are most likely to be associated with abnormal bleeding. Fibroids on the outside of the womb may be associated with a frequent need to urinate, and pain during sex. Many women have fibroids that do not cause any problems. Fibroids usually shrink after the menopause as hormone levels fall. They are more common in certain groups of women (e.g., older women, women with a family history of fibroids, women who are overweight and women of African Caribbean origin).

A polyp is an overgrowth of the lining of the womb, a little like a skin tag elsewhere in the body. They are usually nothing to worry about but can cause problems with bleeding such as heavy bleeding or bleeding between periods.

Endometriosis

Endometriosis is a complex disorder in which tissue that is similar to the lining of the womb (endometrial tissue) is found in other parts of the body (Figure 18). This is most often found on the outside of the womb, in the ovaries, fallopian tubes and in the lining of the peritoneal cavity (which contains the stomach, intestines, liver, spleen and pelvic organs), but it may occur anywhere in the body. The tissue is sensitive to changes in hormone levels, so it builds up and then breaks down and bleeds in association with the menstrual cycle. Pain in the pelvis and other symptoms (such as bloating, diarrhoea, bleeding from the belly button, pain when passing urine or faeces) are usually worse during menstruation. Bleeding may cause inflammation and scarring, causing structures in the body to stick together (called adhesions), and sex may be painful because of this.

It is thought that up to 10% of women have endometriosis, and a significant number of women who have heavy periods are likely to have endometriosis. It can affect women of any age, including younger women. In fact, it has been suggested that, among women with endometriosis, up to 60% started having symptoms before 20 years of age. Up to half of women who struggle to conceive have endometriosis. However, many women who have endometriosis can and do get

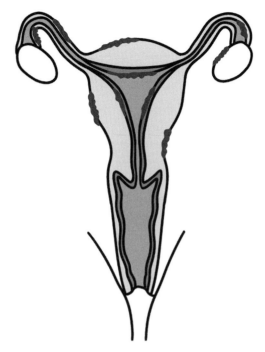

Figure 18 In endometriosis, hormone-sensitive tissue similar to the lining of the womb (endometrial tissue) is found in other parts of the body – usually the outside of the womb, in the ovaries, fallopian tubes and in the lining of the peritoneal cavity. The tissue builds up, breaks down and bleeds in association with the menstrual cycle, causing pain and other symptoms. Artwork © Robin Healy 2022.

pregnant, so contraception is needed to prevent an unplanned pregnancy.

Because the endometrial tissue is sensitive to hormones, hormonal contraception (see Box 7) can help relieve the pain and other symptoms.

Treatment of Heavy Bleeding

Hormonal contraception is an important treatment option to reduce heavy bleeding – whether this is primary HMB or secondary to fibroids,

---

Box 7 Hormonal approaches to the treatment of heavy menstrual bleeding

- Combined hormonal contraception – the pill, the patch or the vaginal ring
- Continuous use (no hormone-free interval) has been shown to work better than cyclical use
- POPs (desogestrel or drospirenone pills are better)
- Progestogen-containing coil (those containing 52 mg levonorgestrel work best)
- Contraceptive injection (sometimes given more often than the recommended 12-week interval)

Box 8 Ways in which hormonal contraception reduces bleeding

- Estrogen prevents the follicles in the ovaries from developing, reducing the level of naturally occurring estrogen in the body
- Progestogens prevent ovulation
- Progestogens and estrogen keep the lining of the womb thinner and less likely to bleed
- Withdrawal bleeds are usually lighter and less painful than periods

---

endometriosis or PCOS. Box 7 lists the different treatment options; Box 8 describes how they reduce bleeding. Hormonal coils that contain 52 mg levonorgestrel are usually the first treatment tried for HMB; however, all hormonal contraception, including progestogen-only methods, reduces bleeding and associated pain.

Whilst HMB usually improves with a single method, more than one may be needed to reduce bleeding to an acceptable level (e.g., the hormonal coil and the pill). Some POPs and the contraceptive injection can stop bleeding altogether, although bleeding may be irregular for the first few months.

Side effects differ with different contraceptive methods, so some women may need to try several options to find the one that works best – there are plenty of options to allow treatment to be tailored to the individual woman. It is wise to check with your healthcare professional whether the treatment provided to manage HMB also provides contraception, as there are other non-contraceptive treatments (e.g., tranexamic acid/mefenamic acid).

Premenstrual Symptoms

Four in ten women experience premenstrual symptoms for a few days before and during their period. Five to eight percent of these women have severe symptoms, referred to as premenstrual dysphoric disorder (or PMDD). Symptoms vary and can be both psychological and physical. Psychological symptoms include depression, anxiety, irritability, loss of confidence and mood swings. Physical symptoms include bloating and breast tenderness.

Some women find that physical premenstrual symptoms improve when they use combined hormonal contraceptive pills that contain certain progestogens (e.g., drospirenone), which reduce fluid retention, minimising breast tenderness and bloating. Taking the pill continuously without a break (hormone-free interval) reduces the risk of breakthrough ovulation.

Acne

Acne in women may be caused by high levels of androgens, which increase the amount of sebum (oil) produced by the skin. Combined hormonal contraceptive pills which contain progestogens that block the androgen receptor (drospirenone and cyproterone acetate) can be used for both contraception and to control acne.

Perimenopausal Symptoms

During the perimenopause – the years leading up to the menopause – ovulation becomes less predictable, and levels of estrogen vary. Without ovulation, there is no progesterone to balance the effect of estrogen on the lining of the womb. The lining can become thick and is shed unpredictably, leading to irregular and often heavy bleeding. HMB is a common but under-recognised symptom of the perimenopause.

Ovulation may continue to occur during the perimenopause but becomes less predictable. It is important to continue using contraception until age 55 years, by which time pregnancy is highly unlikely.

Use of combined hormonal contraception during the perimenopause can help to stabilise hormone levels and also reduce common symptoms of the menopause such as hot flushes, night sweats and poor-quality sleep. Hormone-replacement therapy (HRT) used to reduce peri-menopausal symptoms does not provide contraception. It is therefore important to discuss approaches to HRT and contraception during the menopause with a healthcare professional.

Polycystic Ovary Syndrome

PCOS is a misleading name, because it is associated with unruptured follicles in the ovary, rather than cysts. As these follicles contain eggs that have the potential to develop into a pregnancy if fertilised, contraception is important to avoid an unplanned pregnancy. About 20% of women (one in five) have a polycystic ovary pattern but not the syndrome. For the syndrome, in addition to this type of ovary, women are likely to have heavy if infrequent bleeding and symptoms associated with excess androgens, such as acne and excessive hair growth.

Ovulation is irregular, which means that production of progesterone, which balances the effect of estrogen on the lining of the womb, is lost and the lining can become thick and is shed unpredictably often as a heavy period.

Combined oral contraception that contains the progestogens cypro-terone acetate or drospirenone can help to reduce the symptoms of PCOS caused by high androgen levels (acne and excess hair growth). Progestogen-only contraceptives, particularly the coil, protect the lining of the womb and reduce the risk of HMB in women with PCOS.

Myth busting: Use of hormonal contraception to treat other conditions

Myth 1: I have heavy irregular periods so I can't get pregnant

Fact: A woman may still have ovulated, even if she doesn't have a regular period, so contraception should always be used to avoid an unplanned pregnancy.

Myth 2: I am infertile because I have endometriosis

Fact: While women with endometriosis may struggle to conceive, many do get pregnant, so contraception is needed to prevent an unplanned pregnancy.

Myth 3: The hormonal treatment I am using to help with my gynaecological condition is also providing contraception

Fact: Always confirm with a clinician whether any hormonal treatment you are taking is providing contraception.

Myth 4: HRT provides contraception

Fact: HRT used to relieve perimenopausal symptoms does not provide contraception, other than the Mirena® coil, which may be part of an HRT regimen.

Myth 5: I have heavy periods; I need a hysterectomy

Fact: There are many ways to reduce bleeding, including use of hormonal contraception, non-hormonal medication and endometrial ablation. Few women undergo a hysterectomy nowadays, primarily because of widespread use of the hormonal coil.

INDEX